ANTI-INFLAMMATORY DIET

The Guide for Healing the Immune System, Restoring Your Overall Health and How to Live A Healthy Lifestyle

I0462542

By:

EMY SKYE

CONTENTS

WHY YOU SHOULD READ THIS BOOK

This book is all about inflammation.

Some of our bodies are already on fire on the inside, and some of our habits are the same as throwing petrol on that fire. That's what I will explain today - How to put that fire out, or at least get it back under control.

Just to recap, inflammation is the body's biological response of attempting to protect itself. It aims to remove harmful stimuli, such as pathogens, damaged cells and irritants; this is the first step of the healing process.

Inflammation triggers a response from the immune system. Initially inflammation is beneficial as it is used for protection but a lot of the time inflammation can lead to further inflammation (Chronic) which leads to big health problems.

The five signs to look out for inflammation are pain, redness, heat, swelling and loss of function!

What causes the inflammation in the first place?

- Chronic infections
- Obesity
- Environmental toxins (food, water & air)
- Physiological stress
- Intensive /endurance training
- Physical trauma
- Age
- Autoimmune disease

If you notice that in the brackets for environmental toxins is food. In this book I want to discuss the anti-inflammatory diet. Every food we eat gets a response from the body.

There are certain foods contained in many people's diet today which lead to an increase in inflammation. You can probably guess what kinds of foods these are (fake foods, fried foods, processed foods, refined carbs, coffee, alcohol).

This book talks about what to look for in your life that should either be changed or tweaked toward a lifestyle that is more healthy. We know that there are no solutions to live forever. We can help life a healthier lifestyle to make life more pleasurable.

Cut out foods that cause problems - If you find that you are intolerant to certain foods or you suffer from problems after eating certain foods then cut them out completely. Many people get bad reactions from wheat and gluten containing foods so try cutting out these foods and see if you notice a difference. Eliminate the foods that you suspect cause problems one by one and you will soon uncover the culprit!

INTRODUCTION

Inflammation is a natural process with the biological purpose to initiate healing by increasing circulation. It is a complex process involving both the immune system and vascular system and the interplay of various chemical mediators. Increased circulation brings white blood cells and nourishment to the site of injury or infection so that invading pathogens are killed and damage may be repaired. Characteristic signs of inflammation include pain (dolor), heat (calor), swelling (tumor) and redness (rubor).

Inflammation is the immune systems way of defending against infection and disease. Sometimes your body can be thrown-out-of-balance by the foods we consume, pollutants or the lifestyle you lead.

This can cause the immune system to produce excess inflammation and difficulties will develop. Sometimes these problems start off slowly and are not apparent for several years. Sooner or later inflammation will catch up to you and this will become apparent with problems appearing such as Arthritis.

Besides Arthritis, inflammation can cause cancer,

heart disease, lupus, Alzheimer's and other serious diseases.

As you know drugs have unwanted side effects and can create problems that are worse than what they are treating. There are options such as diet, exercise and supplementation that can help without these side effects.

As with most health problems, inflammation can be brought under control by being in balance with nature. It's clear that the percentage of illnesses today is far greater than past generations. This is due to convenient fast foods, processed food and pollutants in our food and water, as well as all the prescriptions we take for diseases that didn't even exist 50 years ago.

Chronic inflammation is a type of inflammation that silently attacks the body causing disease and degeneration, and is also known as "silent inflammation". As the connection between silent inflammation and a host of diseases becomes clearer, the case for dietary and lifestyle changes that can combat inflammation has become stronger. While it was always known that some conditions such as arthritis and acne were a result of acute inflammation in the body, there is mounting evidence that silent inflammation plays a role in heart disease, Alzheimer's, diabetes and some cancers, as well as in the ageing process. Chronic inflammation can be present undetected in your body for years, until it manifests in disease.

Silent inflammation has been linked with the buildup of cholesterol deposits in the arteries which can lead to heart disease. In a similar way, the risk of Alzheimer's disease increases with inflammation of brain tissue, as this results in the buildup of amyloid plaque deposits in the brain. Having type 2 diabetes, or eating sugary foods contributes to silent inflammation in the body as a result of elevated blood sugar and insulin levels. Recent studies have also confirmed the link between inflammation and several types of cancers. Making the necessary lifestyle changes to fight inflammation, can protect you from it's devastating effects.

There are molecules in the body called prostaglandins which play an important role in inflammation. It has been found that of the three main types of prostaglandins, two of them (PG-E1 and PG-E3) have an anti-inflammatory effect, while the third type (PG-E2) actually promotes inflammation. When there is an imbalance in the body between these prostaglandins, inflammation can result. Prostaglandins are made in the body from essential fatty acids. You can assist your body in making anti-Inflammatory prostaglandins by eating vegetables, nuts, grains and seeds such as sesame and sunflower seeds. On the other hand, foods that cause a spike in insulin levels, such as sugary foods, or foods with a high Glycemic load promote production of PG-E2 and increase inflammation.

A typical anti-inflammatory diet focuses on fighting inflammation through the consumption of foods that lower insulin levels. To actively reduce inflammation, you should therefore eat foods that have a low Glycemic load, such as whole grains, vegetables and lentils, and consume healthy fats such as nuts, seeds, fish, extra virgin olive oil and fish. Spices such as turmeric, ginger, and hot peppers also reduce inflammation. At the same time, you also need to reduce consumption of foods that are pro-inflammatory, such as red meat, egg yolks and shellfish. Sugar is a key culprit in inflammation, and therefore you should also cut back on sugary foods.

Inflammation can also be reduced by taking supplements such as fish oils which are high in Omega 3 fatty acids. When Inflammation Goes Awry:

While some inflammation is beneficial and appropriate for healing, chronic or excessive inflammation, serving no purpose produces damage. Chronic inflammation has a bad reputation because it is implicated in various disease processes including (but not limited to) ...

- autoimmune diseases
- arthritis
- diabetes
- Alzheimer's disease
- atherosclerosis (hardening of arteries that leads to heart attack and stroke)
- ADD and ADHD
- allergies & asthma
- Cancers
- inflammatory bowel disease

Soft tissue swelling and chemical mediators involved in inflammation can also irritate nerve endings, contributing to pain.

Most people who experience inflammation have heard all about the medications that are available to cure the pain and swelling that can occur during a flare up. But how many know that there are some great anti-inflammatory foods that can affect how you feel and reduce the pain associated with inflammation. Following an anti-inflammatory diet will help you beat inflammation naturally.

Inflammation is a swelling that may cause pain, discoloration and even the loss of movement. Usually most people experience severe inflammation when they are the sufferers of arthritis and when they have problems like heart disease and strokes.

Usually your doctor will recommend that you get sleep and exercise in moderation. He may also suggest lowering your weight and taking steroid based drugs or undergoing joint replacement surgery. The medications do work fairly well in reducing the inflammation but often come with some serious side effects, such as ulcers and kidney problems. This may make you wonder if they are worth taking and whether using them is trading one illness for another.

Just like there are some foods that decrease inflammation, there are some that will increase the likelihood that you will get inflammation. These foods are junk foods, fast foods, sugar, and fatty meats. Processed foods that contain Trans and saturated fats also increase the risk of inflammation. Other large contributors of saturated fats are dairy products and eggs. By simply choosing low fat milk, low fat cheese and leaner cuts of meat, you can lower the risks of inflammation, as well as cut down on the chances of chronic disease and obesity. Other foods that increase inflammation include presweetened cereals and soft drinks.

In addition to these, there are foods that are high in sugar and foods that come from the plants labeled as nightshade type. These add to the risk of discomfort associated with inflammation. Eating whole fruits and vegetables will give you the natural healing factors. However, not all vegetables work that way. Potatoes, eggplant and tomatoes can actually make inflammation worse.

So remember the best foods to have are whole fruits, fresh vegetables, lean meats, low fat milk and cheese, as well as fruit and vegetable juices that contain carrots and celery. These types of foods will reduce inflammation and help you get on with your life without pain. Eating right will help you beat inflammation naturally.

CHAPTER 1

CAUSES OF INFLAMMATION

Inflammation is not evil. In fact, it is the result of the body's response to infections and other foreign invaders. The problem starts when there is too much of this going on in the body. What causes inflammation? Here are some examples that you might not even realize.

Inflammation is one thing that happens once the human body's defense mechanisms become active. In which place the defense mechanisms are starting to do their job in your body, it means that place gets to be inflamed. In specific, this problem is triggered by whitened bloodstream cells. Once the body gets to be infected by some outdoors threats the whitened bloodstream cells start to battle and try to eliminate the problem. When whitened bloodstream cells do attack the contamination, they release types of chemicals into the bloodstream. These chemicals may cause the areas of the body to become a little infectious, tender and swell in dimensions.

All these chemicals released in some areas of the

body cause that specific to swell and this is exactly what gives inflammation its looks. Other signs and symptoms of inflammation may include feelings of stiffness or tenderness. For example, when the inflammation is on the part of the body that is responsible with moving an arm, it might hurt to maneuver that part of the body. In some instances, the soreness might be so severe that's it's impossible to maneuver that area of the body for a while.

Another manifestation of inflammation is temperature. Areas of the body which are inflamed will frequently feel totally warm. Areas of the body struggling with inflammation could also appear red-colored in color. Inflammation in your body continues until the agents attacking your body are completely eliminated.

Inflammation is generally categorized in 2 types. First, there's acute inflammation. Acute inflammation is the shorter of these two and it is usually temporary. Second, there's chronic inflammation. This type of inflammation is extremely lasting in time. Actually, it might be a manifestation of a disorder that an individual is affected with for a long time.

Fortunately, you will find there are certain techniques you can use to deal with inflammation. One long-term method an individual can use will be to make some changes in the diet. In specific, use of omega three essential fatty acids can help to eliminate occurrences of inflammation. Omega three essential fatty acids are available in some types of seafood which are full of skin oils, for example fish. These essential fatty acids can be found in some types of nuts, fruits, and veggies too.

A different way to lower occurrences of inflammation would be to somehow reduce the stress level in your life. Stress can release something referred to as cortisol in to the body's bloodstream. This could trigger the defense mechanisms and cause inflammation. Easy methods to lower an individual's stress level include working out, getting enough sleep, and consuming less red-colored meats and fiber.

Certain natural supplements might help effectively to treat inflammation. Included in this are supplements based on silica and zeolite content. Such natural mineral supplements are made to help cleanse your body of certain harmful toxins, for example chemical toxins and environment contaminants. Without such harmful toxins in your body, the defense mechanisms are less needed to be triggered and so, the instances of inflammation will get to be reduced.

Diet. If you frequently experience different forms of inflammation, the first thing you should check is your diet. Here's a look at what causes inflammation through the foods you consume.

• Polyunsaturated vegetable oils - corn, peanut, soy, and sunflower are some examples of oil that are high in their content of linoleic acid, an omega-6 fatty acid. Unlike omega-3 fatty acids that relieve inflammation, omega-6 fatty acids promote inflammation. This is why you need to make sure that you consume a diet that is balanced in omega-3 and omega-6.

• Refined carbohydrates - the inflammation reaction to carbohydrates differs from person to person. Based on research, however, the more the carbohydrate has undergone processing, the faster it is converted to blood glucose and the higher the glycemic index. When the glycemic index is high, the more insulin is released, which is one of the causes of inflammation.

• Red meat - studies have shown that a molecule (sugar found in non-human mammals) become absorbed in the tissues of persons consuming certain types of red meats. Subsequent tests have shown that the presence of this type of sugar (that human are unable to produce genetically) in the body can trigger an immune system response that is one of the inflammation causes.

Then there are other factors that cause inflammation:

• Stress. Whenever we undergo trying situations, the body releases the stress hormone cortisol through the adrenal glands.

Cortisol raises blood pressure and blood sugar levels to help you survive the short bouts of stress. However, its long-term effect is bad.

So, what causes inflammation when a person is stressed? Although cortisol is anti-inflammatory hormone, all it does is suppress parts of the immune system. This means that while cortisol is doing its job, the immune system is unable to fight new infections that affect the body, which can lead to more health problems.

• Environment. Air fresheners, adhesives, glue, cleaning products, pollution, pesticides - these are just some of the chemicals we expose ourselves to everyday. Whether you are in your workplace, on the streets, and even inside your house, there is the possibility that you and your family are not safe from these irritants.

The effect on the immune system differs from person to person because of the varying levels of immunity that everyone has. Nevertheless, constant exposure to these chemicals can someday trigger an immune system response that can lead to inflammation.

• Menopause. There are many changes in a woman's body during menopause. One of which is the loss of hormones that were present in the early stages of life.

Studies have shown that the loss of hormones may

lead to chronic inflammation.

In turn, chronic inflammation has been associated with osteoporosis, cancer, heart disease, and other autoimmune diseases. Furthermore, chronic inflammation causes the body to attack itself. This means that the immune system, which responds to infections, keeps attacking even when there is no longer any danger.

CHAPTER 2

<u>CERTAIN FOODS THAT</u>
<u>CONTRIBUTE TO INFLAMMATION</u>

The list of foods to prevent for that anti-inflammation diet plan includes all wheat products, dairy items, potatoes, tomatoes, corn, sugar, citrus fruits, pork, commercial (nonorganic) eggs, shellfish, peanuts and peanut butter, coffee, alcohol, juice, caffeinated teas, soda, something containing hydrogenated oils, processed meals, and fried foods.

Numerous of these meals can lead directly to irritation. For instance, tomatoes and potatoes, which are component of the Solanaceae or nightshade family of vegetables, are recognized to cause irritation. Tomatoes and potatoes ought to certainly be avoided by anybody with arthritis of any type. Dairy items are worth mentioning because they have a tendency to become very higher in fat.

The amount of weight really isn't the problem, although, because the quantity of fat-soluble poisons which are stored within the weight becomes the true issue. We know that conventionally raised dairy cows, and consequently dairy products, are bombarded with poisons in the form of pesticide residues on feed and genetically modified soy products in the feed.

Many cattle, who are naturally herbivores, are even fed animal protein, which consists of its own accumulated toxins and therefore in turn further increases the total toxin load in dairy products. Like a result, dairy products contribute to the load of toxins that the body's immune program must procedure and get rid of (or store if the body is under tension and thus unable to get rid of the poisons).

You might be wondering how you're going to obtain the calcium necessary for bone health if you're asked to avoid milk. Isn't avoiding milk particularly risky for that development of children's bones? The dairy industry has done an superb job of marketing the notion that everyone needs to drink milk to keep bones wholesome and strong.

In truth, there are many nondairy sources of calcium, including fortified soy, rice, oat, almond, and other nut milks. The entire body absorbs only about 30 percent from the calcium contained in dairy items. The Townsend Letter for Doctors and Individuals, inside a summary of more than twenty various articles, concluded that an allergy to cow's milk is common among adults and kids.

In fact, intact milk proteins are recognized to stimulate the secretion of proinflammatory cytokines in susceptible individuals, such as those with cow's milk allergy.In addition, simply because our regular diet plan is largely made up of animal proteins (such as milk proteins), which are acidic in nature, the entire body removes calcium from the bones to help balance the pH in the gastrointestinal system. If one finds they do not react to dairy and wish to include it in their diet, I suggest eating only natural dairy products.

They don't include the pesticide residues, hormones, and antibiotic residues normal dairy may include. That's simply because the cows are held to higher feeding standards and therefore do not accumulate unnecessary poisons through their diet. Still, even organic dairy items shouldn't be consumed daily. The best-and an frequently overlooked-substitute to drinking milk is drinking water.

I want my patients to drink half their fat in fluid ounces of filtered drinking water daily. (one cup equals eight fluid ounces. Therefore, a person weighing 140 pounds ought to drink seventy fluid ounces of drinking water every day, which works out to about nine cups, or a little over two quarts.)

Drinking filtered water is important simply because it

reduces the toxin load by filtering out unwanted metals for example aluminum and lead, bacteria, hormones, pesticide residues, industrial pollutants, solvents, toxic elements, along with other water-soluble toxins. Liquids to consume as part of the anti-inflammation diet consist of filtered drinking water and herbal teas made with filtered water.

All caffeinated beverages and beverages containing sugar are prevented. Juice is prevented simply because it is really a big source of concentrated sugar, even though it is a natural sugar. Ask yourself if you can eat four oranges in one sitting. If the answer is no, then you ought to not consume an eight-ounce glass of orange juice, which contains the equivalent amount of sugar yet lacks the beneficial fiber content the whole fruit would have.

Alcohol ought to be prevented because it turns into sugar once in the entire body. Coffee along with other caffeinated beverages are very taxing towards the liver due to their toxin load and are taxing towards the adrenal glands because of caffeine's impact on cortisol amounts. The adrenal glands, located on top of the kidneys, are responsible for maintaining energy, generating sex hormones, balancing blood pressure and blood sugar, and moderating the stress response.

If a person's program is already burdened with

physiological or psychological stressors, caffeine will exhaust any stress-moderating resources left within the body. Caffeine also has a detrimental impact on weight loss and can cause anxiety, anger, insomnia, and irritability. Commercial eggs, beef, and pork are included on the list of foods to avoid largely for the exact same reasons that dairy is to become avoided: simply because of the toxin content material and acidifying nature of the animal protein.

Pork and beef are higher in arachidonic acid, which promotes irritation. Some organic beef is allowed but ought to be eaten sparingly. Pork, even natural, is not permitted on this diet plan because of its potential to stimulate an autoimmune response and due to its fat quality. Pigs have very similar protein structures to humans; therefore, consuming pork can improve the chance of cross-reactions within the immune program.

A cross-reaction occurs when the immune program reacts towards the pork proteins which are so comparable to human proteins, simultaneously triggering an immune response against the body's own cells. In his publication The Maker's Diet, Jordan Rubin describes pork as an unclean meat; he compares pork with beef based on the complexity from the two animals' digestive systems. Rubin states that meat from cows is really a "cleaner" meat than pork because of cows' complex digestion (they have four stomach chambers) and because of what cows eat.

Simply because pigs often live in unclean environments, have noncomplex digestion, and will eat something, including their personal young, he considers them to have lower-quality fats, making them a lower-quality food. Studies have shown that the visible weight content in pork is really high in arachidonic acid compared to beef, although the actual meat of pork is lower in arachidonic acid. The anti-inflammatory diet is developed to nourish the entire body on all levels.

Pork is not permitted on this diet plan for more than one reason: because of its high levels of arachidonic acid and because of its potential to create immune-system imbalance. Natural eggs which are free of hormone and pesticide residues and that come from free-range chickens are permitted, but they should not be eaten each and every day due to their animal-protein content.

Sugar causes numerous abnormal reactions within the body and ought to be avoided by all individuals. Sugar depresses the immune program and doesn't provide any nutrients towards the diet plan. Prolonged high-sugar diets lead to higher glucose amounts, higher insulin levels, and high cholesterol amounts, all of which improve heart illness risk, insulin resistance, and diabetes danger.

Shellfish and peanuts are avoided as part of the anti-inflammation diet simply because many individuals have allergies to them. Peanuts also grow an aflatoxin on their surface, which has been shown to improve the incidence of cancer in some individuals; peanuts must be processed carefully to prevent production of this substance. Corn is another common allergen that needs to be avoided.

Conventionally grown corn has often undergone a significant amount of genetic engineering and been subjected to heavy bombardment with pesticides. Wheat is worth discussing, simply because our regular diet plan has gone wheat crazy. Should you want a good perspective on wheat use in today's diet, ask anyone who has celiac illness, that is a disease of gluten intolerance that results in bowel difficulties.

Believe from the typical American family and what they eat on a everyday basis. As mentioned above, one might have cereal, toast, or pancakes for breakfast, a sandwich for lunch, and then pasta or pizza for dinner. The typical family might consume wheat three times every day. Today, wheat isn't what it was a hundred years ago.

Wheat has been greatly genetically modified; furthermore, many nutrients are removed within the refining and processing of wheat. Genetically modifying wheat has elevated its gluten content material to 90 percent, which is extremely irregular. It's possible that the genetic modification of wheat has changed its structure into something our entire body does not recognize as "safe to pass."

Keep in mind that during the elimination and challenge phase of the diet, you might begin to consume these foods again to see if you react to them. For instance, if you reintroduce peanuts and don't react to them in a negative way, you can consume them, but not every day. (Remember that one from the key functions of a wholesome diet is variety.)

Knowing your food reactions is going to be helpful in treating and preventing chronic disease. Interestingly, a person might find that they react to nonorganic corn, but not to organic corn. Finally, besides foods that commonly trigger allergies or sensitivities, other meals that ought to be avoided are processed meals, meals containing hydrogenated oils, and fried foods. Foods containing hydrogenated oils, such as fried meals, stimulate the release from the inflammation promoting prostaglandins.

Any meals that are processed are likely to include big amounts of preservatives, toxins, and dyes, all of which contribute towards the body's overall toxic load. In addition, they have often been sitting on shelves for weeks or months prior to purchase, clearly reducing their level of vital nutrients.

CHAPTER 3

WHO NEEDS AN ANTI-INFLAMMATORY DIET?

Inflammation is often associated with injury. You stub your toe and the toe swells. This is the basic inflammatory reaction. Some people even understand that redness around a cut is also a form of inflammation that the immune system uses to heal the injury. What is not commonly known is the fact that inflammation occurs inside the body as well. When the body exists in an inflammatory state, risk of illness, cancer and heart conditions can increase. An anti-inflammatory diet is an easy way to combat this aftereffect and reduce risk today.

I Don't Suffer From Inflammation!

This is the most common statement and the least correct. Inflammation affects every person in the world at some point in their life. In western cultures, like the United States, a huge portion of the population is affected by inflammation every day. Being overweight or obese is the most common inflammatory condition. It is this inflammatory response that could be the cause of some weight related conditions like diabetes.

When fat cells grow, they take up the free space around the organs. Blood flow can be constricted and the body often feels as though it needs to fight to function normally. When the body feels threatened, inflammation occurs as a natural, healing response. Unfortunately, unlike the small cut that will heal in a few, short days. Obesity takes time to correct and the longer the body lives inflamed, the greater the risk of long term effects.

In the case of obesity, changing the diet by reducing calories will reduce body weight and thus reduce the inflammation in the body. This is the simplest benefit of an anti-inflammatory diet. However, people who are obese or overweight are not the only people who can benefit from an anti-inflammatory diet.

Illness Treatment and Prevention

There are many illnesses and conditions caused by inflammation. These include asthma, arthritis, inflammatory bowel syndrome, pelvic inflammatory disease, endometriosis, diabetes, COPD, Psoriasis, Colitis, and Lupus - just to name a few. All-in-all, there are nearly 40 autoimmune conditions currently accepted by the medical community that are affected by inflammation.

What Can I Do?

The first step is to make dietary changes to reduce food based inflammation. Processed foods, fast foods and prepackaged foods can cause increased inflammation in the body. Replacing these foods with lean meats, whole grains and healthy fats will make a tremendous different in how the body reacts to inflammation. In addition, if weight is a problem, reducing weight while changing to an anti-inflammatory diet can increase the benefits exponentially.

Changing to an anti-inflammatory diet does not have to be in reaction to a disease or illness. Prevention is the best choice and the anti-inflammatory diet can reduce the risk of contracting many of the listed illnesses. When the body feels as though it needs to fight for survival, inflammation occurs, so offering healthy foods that have an inflammatory effect is a great choice for all people including those who are young, healthy and feel they do not need an anti-inflammatory diet.

CHAPTER 4

THE ANTI-INFLAMMATORY DIET: HOW IT CAN PROTECT YOU FROM DISEASE

Inflammation is a good thing. It is the natural way your body responds to threats such as infections or wounds. We have all seen inflammation at work when we have pain and redness at an injury. We say it looks inflamed, and it literally is, because injury activates the inflammatory response.

When is inflammation a problem?

When inflammation lasts for long periods of time, we call it chronic, and it can cause problems. Some common causes of chronic inflammation include allergies, autoimmune disease, periodontal disease, arthritis and other diseases that activate the immune system over time. Even obesity is inflammatory, because fat cells give off chemicals called cytokines that trigger inflammation.

Why is it a problem?

Chronic inflammation causes damage to the endothelial lining of arteries, which can lead to atherosclerosis and heart disease. There is also evidence that it contributes to type 2 diabetes, Alzheimer's disease and a growing number of other chronic diseases that are common in modern, western societies.

What are the symptoms?

The symptoms of inflammation vary with what is causing it. You may even have no symptoms at all, as in the case of obesity. Here are some examples of specific disease related symptoms:

Arthritis, rheumatoid arthritis (joint pain, stiffness, swelling)

Crohn's disease or ulcerative colitis (abdominal pain and cramping, fever, diarrhea) Psoriasis or eczema (redness) Allergies (respiratory symptoms, hives)

More subtle, early indicators of problems could include headaches, muscles aches, fatigue, muscle stiffness, nausea, vomiting, diarrhea or constipation, gas, abdominal discomfort and even emotional problems including depression. These could be related to food sensitivities and intolerances. The most common food intolerances include dairy (lactose), wheat (gluten), yeast, soy, corn, eggs and even some artificial sweeteners.

How can you know if you have chronic inflammation if you don't have symptoms or a diagnosis?

You can find out if you have inflammation by having your C- reactive protein levels tested. The high sensitivity C-reactive protein, is the preferred indicator of chronic, low-grade inflammation.

What should I do if I have high levels of C-reactive protein?

If your C-reactive protein levels are high, you will first want to talk to your doctor to find out if there is an underlying infection, allergy, autoimmune disorder or other contributing disease. If not, your excess weight could be the cause and weight loss is your best line of defense. If you are a smoker, that could also be contributing to the problem.

How do foods influence inflammation?

Inflammation can also be influenced by the foods you eat. Research has shown that certain foods trigger inflammation and others suppress it.

Some of the foods that are pro-inflammatory include:

- Animal fats (corn-fed beef, dark meat and skin of poultry, pork, duck

- Hydrogenated fats (trans fat)
- Fried foods (fried in saturated, hydrogenated or polyunsaturated fats
- Sweets (sugar, candy, cookies, cakes, ice cream, donuts, sweet drinks)
- Refined grains (white bread, pasta, white rice)
- Processed foods (chips, crackers, fries, cold cuts, hot dogs, canned meats)
- Dairy products (especially full fat milk, cheese, sour cream, cream cheese, cream)

Some people may also need to avoid the nightshades (potatoes, tomatoes, eggplant, peppers)

Here are some of the best anti-inflammatory foods:

- Fatty fish such as salmon, sardines, herring, trout and tuna (with omega 3 fatty acids)
- Grass fed beef also contain some omega 3 fats (unlike corn-fed beef, mostly saturated fats)
- Nuts and seeds (walnuts, flaxseed, almonds)
- Monounsaturated fats (olive oil, canola oil, avocados), by replacing polyunsaturated fats
- Turmeric (part of most curry dishes)
- Ginger, used in Asian cuisine (also helps control nausea)
- Whole grains (except wheat, barley and rye if you are gluten intolerant)

Foods that have high antioxidant levels also tend to

reduce inflammation, possibly by reducing the damage that stimulates inflammation. Antioxidants are prolific in brightly and darkly colored fruits and vegetables.

Some of the best sources of antioxidants include:

- Berries: blueberries, raspberries, blackberries, cranberries, strawberries, cherries,
- Beans: Red beans, kidney beans, pinto and black beans
- Herbs: oregano, basil, sage, marjoram, thyme, dill, garlic, dry mustard
- Spices: cinnamon, cloves, cumin, turmeric, ginge
- Nuts: pecans, walnuts, pistachios
- Green tea is rich in both antioxidants and anti-inflammatory compounds
- Coffee, cocoa (or dark chocolate) and red wine (but caffeine and alcohol are inflammatory)
- Exotic fruits: acai, gogi, pomegranate, papaya, pineapple

Eating more of these anti-inflammatory and high antioxidant foods can help calm chronic inflammation and by doing so, reduce your risk for chronic diseases. Find ways to make these foods a part of your everyday diet and you will not only be protecting your body from disease, but you may find that some of your aches and pains improve.

So how do I jump start the anti-inflammatory diet?

Get a journal and write down all the foods you eat in a given week. Think of this first week as a natural eating time, so don't make any changes or eat anything you would not normally eat. Once the list is complete, head off to the Internet for a little research and education on the power of food over inflammation. Many people are surprised by the effects seemingly healthy foods can have on overall body health and the prevention of illness. Sure, the market screams at the consumer about drinking more vitamin C and reducing calories, but what about the foods that seem healthy but really aren't? These foods will be found after a week of journaling before starting your anti-inflammatory diet.

Are there any baked foods on the list? Chances are, if these foods were purchased prepackaged; they will contain at least a small amount of trans fats. Even the small, 100 calorie bites of cupcake marketed as healthy alternatives can contain up to 0.5 grams of trans fats. Eating just two of these little cakes a day for a week contributes a whopping 7 grams of trans fats - the only healthy level is 0 grams.

Did you eat a salad this week? Many people think

eating a salad is a healthy alternative and it can be, without that fat laden dressing covering the healthy greens. One tablespoon of regular dressing can contain 100 calories and about 10 grams of fat. The typical true serving is about ¼ cup per salad. That equates to 400 calories, 40 grams of fat and a -76 rating on the inflammation factor scale which measures the total inflammatory effect of foods on the body. The goal is to reach +50 or more.

Few people look at the foods they eat in an inflammatory way. But, the fact is that many common illnesses that can be life threatening is linked to inflammation. Choosing foods that contain no trans fats and low total fat is a healthy choice toward building your anti-inflammatory response. These changes are simple and anyone can jump onto the diet at any time.

What is the Anti-Inflammatory Diet?

It is a well-known fact that different foods are metabolized differently, some promoting inflammation and others reducing it. The purpose of the anti-inflammatory diet is to promote optimal health and healing by choosing foods that reduce inflammation. If one can successfully control excessive inflammation through natural means (like through diet), it reduces one's dependence on anti-inflammatory medications that have unwanted and unhealthy side effects and don't solve the underlying problem. While anti-inflammatory medications (such as NSAIDs) are a quick fix to ease symptoms, they ultimately weaken the immune system by damaging the gastrointestinal tract which plays an important role in immune system function (1).

Anti-inflammatory Diet Basics:

In general, eat an abundance of fresh vegetables and fruits, whole grains, anti-inflammatory fats and nuts while limiting processed foods, meat protein, milk products, refined sugars, artificial colors/flavors/sweeteners and food sensitivities.

Vegetables:

Eat and Enjoy: Enjoy an abundance of fresh vegetables and fruits in a variety of colors (preferably organic). Fruits and vegetables are full of vitamins, minerals, antioxidants and fiber which give the body the essential building blocks for health. Examples include beans, squash, lintels, sweet potatoes, cruciferous vegetables, avocados, dark leafy greens... There are so many choices! As for fruits, pineapple and papaya are particularly good because they are high in bromelain, a powerful natural anti-inflammatory. Fruits and vegetables also make great, healthy snacks.

Avoid / Limit: Avoid produce that is not grown

organically. Toxic chemical residues from herbicides and pesticides can remain and when ingested are foreign irritants to the system. Many crops in North America are also genetically engineered and are put on the market without rigorous scientific study to determine safety for human consumption. Independent research is finally being done to show toxic effects of consuming genetically modified organisms (2). Foreign DNA is randomly inserted into the genome of a crop. Examples include herbicide resistant corn and soy which are resistant to the herbicide Roundup, made by Monsanto. Roughly 90% of all corn and soy sold in North America is genetically modified. Also be aware of derivatives of genetically modified ingredients (such as corn starch and corn syrup etc.). It has also been suggested that consuming GMOs is a contributing factor to the rise in allergies as our bodies are recognizing these food substances as foreign (3). By choosing items with the "certified organic" label, you avoid both GMOs and toxic herbicides/pesticides.

For some people, vegetables in the nightshade family may pose a concern. Examples of nightshade vegetables include tomatoes, peppers, potatoes and eggplant. Nightshades contain alkaloids which are thought to exacerbate inflammation and joint damage in certain susceptible individuals with arthritis (though research is conflicting). Thus, for some individuals, limiting or avoiding nightshade vegetables may be beneficial.

Fats:

Eat and Enjoy: Enjoy healthy, anti-inflammatory fats including olive oil, coconut oil, avocados, nuts, salmon and sardines. In humans, there are two essential fatty acids, alpha-linolenic acid (an omega-3) and linoleic acid (an omega-6). These are "essential" because they are required for good health but the body does not synthesize them. Omega-3 fats are anti-inflammatory. Omega-6 fats can be pro-inflammatory or anti-inflammatory (as it can be metabolized by two different pathways). Researchers suggest that keeping the ratio of omega-6 to omega-3 between 2:1 and 4:1 is best for health. The modern diet tends to be high in omega-6 as it is abundantly available in cooking oils. Thus, including rich sources of omega-3 is important (such as fish, flax and walnuts especially). Avoid / Limit: Fats to limit or avoid include margarine, butter, shortening, hydrogenated oils, trans fats, saturated fats, and milk fat. Omega-6 fats are very high in corn oil, safflower oil and sunflower oil. Trans fats are linked with inflammatory diseases.

Meat:

Eat and Enjoy: In general, limit animal proteins because they tend to acidify the body and also promote inflammation. When selecting animal protein, enjoy fish, poultry (especially free-range and organically raised), lamb and omega-3 eggs.

Avoid / Limit: Limit beef, pork, shellfish and factory farmed eggs. In general, grass-fed is superior to grain-fed. Avoid charred foods, smoked foods and cold cuts. Cold cuts contain nitrates and nitrites which promote cancer. Barbequed foods contain polycyclic aromatic hydrocarbons (PAHs) and heterocyclic amines (HCAs) which also promote cancer.

Dairy:

Eat and Enjoy: Enjoy dairy substitutes in moderation (such as almond milk).

Avoid / Limit: Avoid or limit dairy products in general. This includes milk, yogurt, cheese and ice cream. As we age, we lose the enzyme that digests dairy, resulting in lactose intolerance and inflammation. The milk protein, casein, is also acidifying which (despite what many people are brought up thinking) robs the bones of calcium.

Grains:

Eat and Enjoy: Enjoy whole grains as opposed to refined grains. Refined grains are grains in which the germ and bran have been removed. This means there is loss of fiber, minerals and vitamins. In other words, the good stuff is removed in exchange for a longer shelf life. Some good examples of healthy grains include (organic) whole wheat/oats/bulgar/coucous, quinoa and whole oats (like steel-cut oats).

Whole grains are also a rich source of complex carbohydrates. Complex carbohydrates (as opposed to simple sugars) will prevent spikes in your blood sugar level. Sugar promotes inflammation.

Avoid / Limit: Avoid or limit refined carbohydrates such as white bread, pastries, sweet things and pastas.

Nuts:

Eat and Enjoy: Enjoy nuts and nut butters such as almonds, walnuts, sesame seeds, pumpkin seeds and flax.

Avoid / Limit: Avoid any specific nut allergies.

Beverages:

Eat and Enjoy: Enjoy plenty of pure, filtered water (avoiding chlorine, fluoride and other contaminants which are irritants that promote inflammation). Other great choices are lemon water and herbal teas.

Avoid / Limit: Avoid sugary sodas, fruit juice (with sugar added) and milk.

Spices:

Eat and Enjoy: Many spices reduce inflammation. Some great examples are turmeric, oregano, rosemary, ginger, garlic and cinnamon. Bioflavenoids and polyphenols reduce inflammation and fight free radicals. Cayenne pepper is also anti-inflammatory, as it contains capsicum. Capsicum is often used in pain-relief creams.

Sweeteners:

Eat and Enjoy: Enjoy stevia, molasses, maple syrup or honey as better alternatives for refined sugar.

Avoid / Limit: Avoid refined sugar, fructose and especially high fructose corn syrup which promote inflammation. Avoid artificial sweeteners.

Other:

Eat and Enjoy: fermented foods such as kimchi, miso soup and sauerkraut. Fermented foods are probiotic and help to rebuild the immune system by supporting healthy microflora in the gut and to reduce inflammation. Fermented foods also tend to be easy to digest and are also factories for B vitamins.

Avoid / Limit: In general, eliminate processed foods, artificial colors, artificial flavors and preservatives. Also, avoid foods that you have a known sensitivity or allergy to as this promotes inflammation. Low grade sensitivities are easy to miss, so if you're unsure, have a food allergy test. Some of the most common problem foods include wheat (gluten), corn, soy, milk and nuts.

CHAPTER 5

THE COMPLETE GUIDE FOR HEALING IMMUNE SYSTEM

Optimal health means more than the absence of pain, sickness and disease. As important as it is to be physical healthy it is equally important to be mentally, emotionally and spiritually healthy as well. Optimal health, therefore, in context of what is being written here, is a balance of physical, mental, emotional, and spiritual aspects of health. Let us take a look at each of these aspects, beginning with physical health.

So much has been written about the subject of physical health in the categories of health and wellness, diet and weight loss, fitness and bodybuilding etc. In this article I will primarily deal with physical health in its internal aspect which includes building a healthy immune system, detoxifying the body, healthy and quick elimination, and nourishing the cells with proper nutrition. Aging itself can be slowed down by keeping the internal aspect of our physical health up to par. Wouldn't you love to have a healthy, youthful, energetic, strong, lean body which is free of disease, sickness and pain well into adulthood beyond the age of 40? It all narrows down to what type of food we put into our bodies - either food filled with toxins and poisons, or healthy, living, vital food.

Food is intended to furnish the body with all the live elements needed for the regeneration of its cells and tissues. If the body fails to be healthy, the lack or deficiency of regenerative elements in the food is the cause of, and the responsibility for, whatever ailment, sickness or disease overtakes it. Our bodies seek homeostasis, equilibrium, balance. This equals health. When given the right building blocks to work with, the body maintains itself in health.

Super-foods are known to:

Deter Aging

Massively Boost Your Immune System

Aid Weight Loss

Lower Your Cholesterol

Radically Improve Your Energy

Enhance Your Mental & Emotional Well-being

Boost Your Libido

Alkalize Your System

Protect against Toxins and Pollutants

Beautify Your Skin

Cleanse and Fortify Your Blood

Nourish and Revitalize your Systems

Fight and Protect against numerous diseases including Diabetes, Hypertension, Heart Disease, Stroke, Cancer, Arthritis, Cataracts, Osteoporosis, Acne, Obesity, High cholesterol, Age-Related Blindness...And Much More!

Basically if we put the wrong food (and drink) into our body it weakens the immune system and opens the door for us to be susceptible to health problems of whatever sort (whether it be frequents colds and sicknesses, flues, aches and pains, sores and ulcers, weakness, sluggishness, high blood pressure, high cholesterol, arthritis, heart problems, diabetes, cancer or psychological disorders such as malaise, apathy or memory problems etc., etc., etc.) Looking on the bright side a healthy immune system that is not swamped with toxins can fight off diseases successfully!

It is preferable to never be unhealthy to begin with and to eat nothing but healthy food from day one. Unfortunately, it is not this way. Many have been conditioned to eat unhealthy, fattening, artery clogging foods from childhood to the grave. Many of us think it is a normal part of the aging process to start getting weaker, fatter, having more pain etc. after age 30 and onward. In many cases (definitely not all) premature aging and bodily weakening is the result of years of poor eating habits from childhood to adulthood. Due to many years of wrong eating habits it may be best to detoxify.

In the process of nourishing our cells with foods high in fiber such as vegetables, fruits, super-foods, and whole grains our body naturally detoxifies itself in the process, which in turn strengthens our immune system and slows, or in some cases, reverses the aging process. The key to optimal health as far as the physical aspect of our health goes, is to:

Eat plenty of Grains, vegetables, fruits, nuts, super-foods, herbs, being sure to get plenty of exercise, pure water and clean air, excreting waste from the intestines quickly (which is a byproduct of eating plenty of fruits, fiber and vegetables). There are also natural supplements you can take such as Vitamin C, vitamins and minerals, and various antioxidants unless you are getting plenty of these from your regular diet.

I left out other important factors which contribute to overall optimal health. They included, but are not limited to, being healed of emotional traumas, maintaining a calm mental attitude, living in a spirit of prayer, faith, hope and love towards others in general, and towards God, Spirit, Higher Power in particular.

Next, I hope to share a little about the three remaining categories of health - mental, emotional and spiritual.

Mental and Emotional Health

Mental and emotional health are so closely related it is hard to separate the two. Having a healthy mind is not limited to having a keen intellect and an excellent memory. Someone can excel at this level of mental health but still be an emotional wreck, not to mention being spiritually ignorant at the same time.

Negative mental attitudes or emotions can have a direct effect on our physical health even if we are eating healthy food. Emotional traumas, anger, rage, hate, stress etc., when persisted in day in and day out, weaken the immune system and manifest in ill physical health. A negative mind, over time, often erases all the good that healthy food does for us.

Some forms of sickness, disease, and illness, as well as bad habits like smoking, drinking, drugs etc., are often external symptoms of something deeper. They are effects of a deeper cause. And until that cause is addressed and healed the symptoms will keep coming back like fruit on a tree whether in the form of ill health, disease, anxiety, bad habits of one sort or another, or in the worst case scenario cancer. Luckily there are warning signs when all is not well within.

The subconscious part of our mind is the storehouse of our emotions and memories and it is here where we need healing as far as our mental and emotional life are concerned. Sometimes negative or uneasy dreams (some of which originate from the sub conscious) are manifestations of our own fears and internal wounds. Some dreams are also messages, clothed with images we can comprehend, from our highest level of mind - the super conscious level - warning us when we are making wrong decisions, or heading in a wrong direction. In those rare cases where we are susceptible to the healing energies of the super conscious level of mind we can experience internal healing quicker than we ever imagined. More about this in a minute when I get to the spiritual aspect of health.

Along with a healthy diet it is important to think positive thoughts and maintain a positive attitude, avoiding anger and bitterness towards others. But, thinking positive thoughts and making an effort to be happy, loving, and optimistic, are only part of what is involved when it comes to the healing of our emotional life. We can only go so far by exercising will power alone, as important as it is to use our own efforts when attempting to make a change in our emotional life for the better. All our ethical standards, our rules and regulations for leading an acceptable moral life, all our positive thinking formula are a means to an end, the end being the opening and revelation of the spiritual aspect or our mind - the super conscious level of mind. This brings me to the last category of health, the spiritual category.

This is sad and indeed very unfortunate. With so much pollution, tension and stress taking their toll on our health, the one thing that we can do to battle this is to have a nutrition rich anti inflammation diet.

Pollution causes free radical damage and also has serious inflammatory effects which have tremendous adverse effects on our health, leading to numerous ailments including psoriasis, cancer, auto immune diseases, Alzheimer's disease, heart diseases etc.

Can an anti-inflammation diet help here? Of course it can. In fact that is one of the best ways to come out victorious from this maze of diseases and disorders.

An anti- inflammation diet should strictly consist of omega 3 fatty acids which have amazing anti-inflammatory properties. These fatty acids are essentially comprised of DHA (Docosahexanoic Acid) and EPA (Eicosapentaenoic Acid) fats.

Our body internally converts DHA into a substance called Resolvin D2 which is a potent and effective anti-inflammatory agent. It works by inhibiting the production of pro-inflammatory eicosanoids which reduce the inflammation significantly and provide instant relief from various ailments including the common ones like arthritis and gout.

If you want to make this beneficial fatty acid a part of your daily diet, one best and efficient way is to incorporate premium fish oil supplements in your health regimen. Make sure to choose the one having more DHA content than EPA.

This not only helps in ensuring the anti-inflammatory properties contained in DHA but also ensures ample supply of both DHA and EPA to the body. This is due to our body's ability to convert DHA into EPA as per its requirement. Since the reverse reaction is difficult to attain, it is advisable to take a supplement containing more DHA content.

These supplements not only regularize and assure your receiving an anti-inflammation diet, it also ensures that you take it in optimal amounts. The good supplements have the optimal usage per serving specified on them which is one thing to be checked before choosing to incorporate them in your daily regimen.

We are taught from a young age to have an implicit co-dependent relationship with a medical doctor. A person sits with a physician and says, "Doc, here are my symptoms--give me something to fix it."

Although, this is irrational, it is so pervasive that Homeopathic and Naturopathic doctors have taken on this omnipotent and obviously impossible role as well. It is especially true when the person needs to be an active participant in the healing process. People's want/demand for a 'quick fix' and demand that someone 'fix it,' is so pervasive that Homeopaths and Naturopaths have unwittingly taken on this impossible role without realizing the negative outcome. Homeopaths and Naturopaths need to go back to their roots of being co-creators in the healing process--not the omnipotent healer.

Cancer, the most feared disease and the disease, which needs the most work on the part of the person, has the greatest need for co-healers. Holistic health care providers need to educate their clients that cancer or any dis-ease is not 'the enemy,' but rather the consequence of continued violations of natural laws. Because our environment is artificial and we interact with machines rather than nature, we have all but forgotten our bodies are governed by natural laws. Unlike human laws, natural laws are non-negotiable. Suffice to say, planting an orange seed will not yield a pear tree; continued violations of the laws which govern your biology will not yield a healthy body.

The true definition of health is the optimal

functioning of an organism. Health is not, as commonly defined by Traditional Western Medicine (TWM), the absence of disease. The absence of disease is like saying that 'darkness' is the absence of 'light.' Health is the outcome of healthy living. A plan for the restoration of health that is not based on the laws of nature is destined not only to fail, but to disappoint all who follow it.

The immune system has two major functions--the 'department of defense' and the 'department of maintenance.' When overwhelmed by maintenance requirements--cleaning/repair--the immune system has too few resources left for defense, thus, the development of infections, degenerative diseases, such as, cancer can take hold.

A complete holistic approach to healing cancer includes:

 Learning why the person created the cancer. The metaphysical cause of cancer is Deep hurt. Longstanding resentment. Deep secret or grief eating away at the self. Carrying hatreds. A belief--'What's the use?' What issue was the cancer created to revolve? What truth does the cancer want the person to know? Healing and resolving these issues on a mind, body, spirit level is imperative.

The cancer needs to be specifically addressed as a temporary solution rather than 'an enemy.'

The immune system needs to be balanced and enhanced. In order for the body to cease being the messenger, metabolic wastes need to be removed through cleansing the colon, skin and internal organs--Homeopathy, botanicals, exercise, fasting and oxidative therapies.

It is imperative that the nourishment taken in be guided by natural laws and not emotions or deleterious habits. Fresh organic dense nutrient foods that have not been damaged by processing are imperative.

Other modalities can be selectively chosen without destroying the person's healthy cells:

Such as:

1. Insulin Potentiation Therapy
2. High dose intravenous vitamin C
3. Poly MVA

The relationship between healer and the person seeking health is sacred. These relationships define the 'soil' in which health can emerge and blossom. In TWM, the relationship between doctor and patient involves the patient 'handing over' to the doctor their 'disease' and hence the responsibility for its resolution. This implicit pre-conditioned contract is doomed to failure because it is based upon fallacious reasoning and false premises. If the patient is asked to step out of the 'treating symptoms paradigm' and commit to undertaking the journey towards health, healing begins.

The power to heal resides within every living organism and not in anything extrinsic to them. The body is designed to heal itself provided it has the proper emotional, spiritual, nutritional, vitamin and mineral supplement support. Healing is a natural, integral and continuous function of living. We need only to restore those conditions necessary for the natural laws to function unimpeded and healing will prevail over disease and other influences.

The body's immune system is a complex and precise function that recognizes any foreign invasion by any substance, bacteria or virus that will cause disease or harm the host in any way. When a foreign substance invades the body, an inflammatory condition results in the tissues affected. A prime example would be when a patient has tissue transplanted from another person, living or dead into to their body. Their immune system will reject the implanted tissue, and in order to prevent this, they will have to be on specific medications for the rest of their life to try to prevent this rejection.

your immune system is your front line of defense against all invaders to keep you healthy. "Invaders" include pathogens, bacteria, fungi, parasites, and viruses. Collectively, these make up a group of antigens. The response to these is invaders is called the antigen response. The word comes from the generation of antibodies to fight them off.

This sophisticated system is made up of proteins, cells, organs, and tissues. These all interact in a very sophisticated network of partnership towards one goal - keeping you healthy.

To make it simpler, we will refer to all invaders as "the bad guys." The cells and tissues that are normal and healthy, part of your "self", are "the good guys." At any given time, we have lots of these foreign invaders in our body. And we are constantly taking new "bad guys" in through our food, air and water. This defensive system has a tall order to fill, and a healthy immune system never takes a break.

To function properly, it must be able to decide whether or not what enters the body is a good guy or a bad guy. In a properly functioning immune system, the friends and foes are identified correctly. To make matters more complicated, pathogens or "bad guys" can adapt and change quickly, fooling or tricking this system into accepting them, and then you can become sick. So, it's war between the good guys and the bad guys!

When a pathogen enters the bloodstream, there is an immune response. The large white blood cells engulf the pathogens and eat them up. The smaller lymphocytes have to be a little more clever - they have to adapt a specific defense to them. The B Cells identify pathogens as bad guys, then the Killer-T cells kill them. Helper-T cells help out, and when the carnage is over, suppressor T-Cells turn off the immune response.

When it comes to immunity, there is a delicate balance to be maintained. If the immune system is too weak, referred to as Immunodeficiency, or too strong, as in auto-immune disorders, problems can result. Immunodeficiency occurs when a person's immune system is not strong enough to fight off infection. One of the best known examples of immunodeficiency is HIV.

By contrast, an overactive system is referred to as an auto immune disorder or autoimmunity. Here, the normal cells and tissues are identified as enemies, and then the killers (T-cells) and eaters (White Blood Cells) go in and destroy this healthy tissue. Some examples of autoimmune disorders are Rheumatoid Arthritis, Chronic Fatigue Syndrome, Lou Gehrig's Disease, and Lupus.

The immune system you are born with is called your innate immune system. The things that we do to increase our resistance to disease, is part of what is called our adaptive immune system. An example of adaptive immunity is receiving a vaccination, so that your body builds up a defense or antibodies to the vaccine. As a result, if and when you are exposed to the virus that was in the vaccine, your immune system will fight it off and you won't get sick. In this way your immune system has memory.

The study of all aspects of this and how it relates to human health is called immunology. This is an ever growing field, and with complexities that are continually uncovered each day, we learn more about how we can protect ourselves and our health through better understanding of our immune system, both innate and adaptive.

Genes play their part, and we can do the rest. This is our front line of defense against all foreign invaders, so we can certainly strengthen our army of good guys to keep out the bad guys.

In order to do this, it is important to exercise regularly, eat well, get regular rest, maintain a healthy body weight, and supplement with what is missing. It is also important to avoid ingesting toxins wherever possible, and where it is not possible, to eliminate them as soon as they are ingested. And it goes without saying that smoking, alcohol abuse, and inappropriate drug use will do harm to this complex system as well.

Often, when our immunity is down and we get sick, we go to the doctor. At this point the approach is reactive. We are finding more and better ways now to be pro-active, and to prevent this in the first place by stopping the invaders in their tracks. This is done by building a very strong defense - a healthy immune system.

Glutathione has been shown to optimize the adaptive immune system, and so it is very important to boost glutathione levels in order to stay healthy and ward off illness. Glutathione is a balancer, so if you are immune-deficient, you will get stronger. If you have an autoimmune disorder, glutathione will re-balance it.

It "knows" what to do, and gets busy doing it.

Keeping Your Immune System Healthy

A healthy immune system means a overall healthy body. The only way to keep up the best health is to keeping the immune system carrying out properly. This isn't always an easy thing to do with the environment we live in know. The current diet most people are on these days doesn't consist of many vitamins, minerals, antioxidants and other nutritive issues that are necessary to the body to keep up a healthy immune. If your immune system is straining and not at it's finest, we are much more vulnerable to illness.

Having a weak immune system may make you feel

run down and fatigued most of the time, also you catch colds and viruses often, and you're constantly sick. Have you ever noticed how some people catch everything that everyone else has and others are never sick and always full with energy? Different people have different immune systems. Our immune is how we fight off infections, germs and cancer. Some people's immune systems are weaker and don't work properly, as with immunodeficiency disorders. These people are at a big risk to infection and cancer.

The immune function consists of white blood cells, amino acids and some bigger organs. The immune system is multifaceted and important to our healthy being. A strong and balanced immune is necessary for health maintenance. The immune system is composed of many mutually dependent cell types that together protect the body from bacterial, parasitic, fungal and viral infections, as well as from the growth of tumor cells. Many of these cell types have particular functions. The cells of the immune can defeat bacteria, kill parasites or tumor cells, or kill virus infected cells.

The immune system replys can be low by a variety of outside influences including emotional stress, physical stressors such as insufficient sleep or athletic overtraining, environmental and occupational chemical exposure, UV and other types of radiation, common viral or bacterial infections, certain drug therapies, blood transfusions and surgery. Dietary lifestyles also have an impact. Excessive fat, alcohol or refined sugar consumption or not enough of protein, calorie, vitamins, mineral or water intake furthers decreased immune performance as well.

Some ways to avoiding having a weak immune system is wash your hands constantly, one of the easiest ways to pick up germs is through touching something or someone, avoid crowded areas during cold and flu time, take your vitamins every day, people who get sick a lot are often missing main vitamins that they need, keep your areas clean such as your house, office, desk, and also treat all little cuts, even little cuts can be a big thing to people who can't fight germs.

Because of the lack the immune doesn't always show itself in obvious ways, damaged immune function and its exact main cause often avoid detection. It can appear as a genetic or obtain immunodeficiency, or as a temporary or permanent state of depressed immune function due to other problems. Either way, the level of reduced immune ability to respond to pathogenic organisms, tumors or tissue damage is dependent on the environment of the condition, which components of the immune system are affected.

All of the daily stress, infections and disease, our immune systems are compromised, overburdened, and irritated to help keeping all of these way, try ImmuneCea. This formula balances and strengthens the different parts of the immune system with special herb and mushroom extracts.

CHAPTER 6

A HEALTHY IMMUNE SYSTEM EQUALS A HEALTHY YOU

Your immune system is made up of a network of cells, tissues, and organs that work together to protect the body and it appears even in the most structurally-simple forms of life, with bacteria using a unique defense mechanism, called the restriction modification system to protect themselves from viral pathogens, called bacteriophages. Disorders occur when the immune response is inappropriate, excessive, or lacking. Fortunately for most of us, this system is constantly on call to do battle with bugs that could put us out of commission.

This system has a series of dual natures, the most important of which is self/non-self-recognition. Each cell in our body has an antigen that tells the immune system that it is part of us and should not be eliminated. It is through antigens that the our system knows which cells to attack and which to leave alone. Sometimes the process breaks down and attacks self-cells. This is the case of autoimmune diseases like multiple sclerosis, systemic lupus erythematous, and some forms of arthritis and diabetes.

The innate immune system is the dominant system of host defense in most organisms. This comprises the cells and mechanisms that defend the host from infection by other organisms, in a non-specific manner. This means that the cells of the innate system recognize, and respond to, pathogens in a generic way, but unlike the adaptive immune system, it does not confer long-lasting or protective immunity to the host. [18] Innate immune defenses are non-specific, meaning these systems respond to pathogens in a generic way. Natural killer cells, or NK cells, are a component of the innate immune system.

Both innate and adaptive immunity depend on the ability of the immune system to distinguish between self and non-self-molecules. Helper T cells regulate both the innate and adaptive immune responses and help determine which types of immune responses the body will make to a particular pathogen. Adaptive immune responses are actually reactions of the immune system to structures on the surface of the invading organism called antigens.

One of the drawbacks of chemotherapy treatment for cancer, for example, is that it not only attacks cancer cells, but other fast-growing, healthy cells, including those found in the bone marrow and other parts of the immune system. In cancer cells, genetic changes cause changes in the cell-surface antigens such that the person's immune system (hopefully) no longer recognizes them as "self" and destroys them. Boosting the immune system has been shown to be therapeutically valuable in treating a wide variety of cancers, chronic viral infections and other illnesses. Some cells of the immune system can recognize cancer cells as abnormal and kill them. But some new treatments aim to use the immune system to fight cancer.

Another important role of this wonderous system is to identify and eliminate tumors. These antigens appear foreign, and their presence causes immune cells to attack the transformed tumor cells. The main response of the immune system to tumors is to destroy the abnormal cells using killer T cells, sometimes with the assistance of helper T cells. Clearly, some tumors evade the immune system and go on to become cancers. However, if the immune system is stressed and not functioning properly, a cancer cell may multiply before the immune system has a chance to kill it.

The immune system is complex, intricate and interesting. To understand the power of this system, all that you have to do is look at what happens to anything once it dies. That sounds gross, but it does show you something very important about your immune system. Although the immune system is extremely complex, its basic strategy is simple: to recognize the enemy, mobilize forces, and attack. It is under assault from herbicides, pesticides and food additives, and also from the immense amount of radiation that is part of our everyday life today. Protect your immune system and you will live a long healthy life.

Everyone has an immune system, you are born with it. The stronger your immune system the healthier you are. With a strong immune system your body will fight against diseases and illnesses. Your immune system is made up of cells, tissues, proteins, and organs, and it defends people against germs and bacteria every day. In most cases, the immune system does a great job of keeping people healthy and preventing infections. But sometimes problems with the immune system can lead to illness and infection.

What does your immune system do? It is the body's defense against infectious organisms and other viruses. The immune response is the steps your system takes to attack foreign substances in your body, and recovers from infections.

There are many factors that contribute to having strong immunity. Stress will cause your immune system to be low. Daily exercise can boost your immunity, and eating a well-balanced diet will have a great effect on the immune system. Keeping your meals nutritious and healthy is one of the greatest factors of having tough immunity.

The foreign substance that invades your body is called an antigen. When your body detects an antigen the cells work together and recognize the foreign substance and respond to it. These cells activate the B lymphocytes to create antibodies, particular proteins that fasten onto specific antigens. Antibodies' job is to neutralize foreign substances and activate an assembly of proteins called complement. These proteins assist in the process of getting rid of infected cells, or bacteria.

Although antibodies can recognize an antigen and lock onto it, they are not capable of destroying it without help. That is the job of the T cells. These cells are also called killer cells. The T cells attack the infected cells and also signal other cells such as phagocytes to attack and kill as well. The process of all these cells working together is immunity.

There are three types of immunity: innate, passive, and adaptive. Innate immunity refers to the external barricade such as the skin, and mucous membranes found in the nose, throat, and gastrointestinal tract. This wall is broken when a person gets a cut. The skin and its cells will try to heal the cut and attack germs right away. Passive immunity comes from outside sources such as a mother's breast milk. Infants get this immunity when they are young because their immune system is not as strong. It is, however, temporary and won't last the child's whole life. The third type of immunity is adaptive or active immunity. This is the type that develops throughout life. As children and adults are more exposed to certain bacteria, they can develop immunity to those bacteria. Vaccinations allow a small amount of a disease to be put into the body so the immune system can react and build immunity to that disease.

All immune systems are different. Some people get sick all the time, for others it seems that they never get ill. Immune systems tend to become stronger as people get older and are more exposed to certain germs. This is because their immune system has learned to recognize and instantly attack cold-causing germs, bacteria, and viruses. Boosting your immune system with Alligin by Liberty Health can help strengthen your immunity with one of the most powerful broad-range antimicrobial ingredients and keep you healthy and antigen-free!

CHAPTER 7

HOW TO BOOST THE IMMUNE SYSTEM USING HYPNOSIS

Whether or not you realize it, immune system help needs to be your number one priority if you want to live a long and healthy life. The good news is that there are more tools today to boost immunity than at any other time in the past. It is up to you though, to put these tools to work for you.

The Importance of the Immune System

This system is your body's first line of defense against infection and disease. A healthy immune system can fend off many illnesses that have the potential to be lethal. It can also aid in warding off the worst effects of many fatal illnesses. Some people have a natural immunity that is more robust than others. If you need immune system help there are a few options available to help you boost immunity.

Your immune system is one of the most important systems in your body. It protects you from dozens of different diseases, and it does this by fighting off large numbers of bacteria, viruses, fungi and other pathogens that attack your body every day. Furthermore, it also works to stop the initiation of cancer.

Germs are all around us, and if we weren't protected by our immune system, we would be dead in twenty-four hours. It is a complex, sophisticated, and a well organized system, and it has to be kept in top shape if you are to be fully protected. Some of the things that affect it adversely are:

- Improper nutrition
- Stress
- Overweight
- High fat diet
- Little or no exercise
- Not enough sleep
- Smoking
- Environmental toxins
- Some drugs

The white cells in your body (also known as leukocytes) are a major part of your immune system. Most are born in the marrow of your body's long bones. Some of them migrate to the thymus gland early on where they become T-cells. (The thymus is located just above the heart in the chest.) Others remain in the bone marrow, and some of them become what are called B-cells. Together, the T and B cells are referred to as lymphocytes.

While the T-cells are in the thymus they are trained to recognize over a million different antigens, with each T-cell recognizing only one specific antigen. An antigen is a molecular recognition code that is on the surface of all cells; is can be friendly or foreign. If unfriendly, such as those on viruses, it will be attacked. In most cases, however, immune system cells have to be given permission before they can attack. This is because several friendly pathogens live and perform important functions in the body. A good example is the friendly bacteria in your colon that help digest food.

Your thymus works hard to educate billions of T-cells throughout your younger years. As you grow older, however, it begins to shrink in size, and gives you less protection. That's why older people (over about 65) are more susceptible to infections and cancer.

As T-cells mature in the thymus, they take on one of four functions. They can become:

1. Helper T-cells (T-4 cells): These cells are particularly important shortly after the infection occurs. They sound the alarm, and alert the immune system, and they oversee the immune system's response. They are usually activated after particles called macrophages

detect antigens; these macrophages give off cytokines, or messengers, that tell other lymphocytes to begin the attack.

2. Suppressor T-cells (T-8 cells): Once the immune system cells are sent out to fight the antigens, they must be regulated and controlled, particularly after the invaders have been defeated. If not they can attack healthy cells of the body, which may lead to autoimmune disease. Suppressor cells shut down the response when needed.

3. Killer T-cells: These cells kill by injecting poison into the cells containing the antigen. They cannot attack these cells, however, without permission from helper T-cells.

4. Natural Killer cells (NK's): They are primitive T-cells that are free to attack antigens without permission from helper T's. Basically, they are the first line of defense. Targets for them are usually identified by macrophages.

While the war between immune system cells and antigens is going on, it's important for the immune cells to be able to communicate with one another. This is done using hormone-like messengers called cytokines. One of the most important cytokines is interferon. It is released by both T-cells and macrophages, and it guides NK killers to the appropriate targets. It is also used to stop viruses from multiplying, and is helpful in impeding the development of cancer cells.

B-Cells, Antibodies, and Complement :So far we have barely mentioned the B-cells, but they also play a critical role in the war against the antigens. In particular they manufacture antibodies that attack the antigens directly. The B-cells remain in the bone marrow where they eventually become specific for many different antigens. When they mature they move to the body's lymph nodes.

When T-4 cells see a B-cell displaying the antigen of an invader, they authorize the B-cells to produce antibodies against it. The B-cells immediately begin to grow and divide into a large number of plasma cells. These plasma cells are the factories that produce antibodies. Within a few days each B-cell divides into hundreds of plasma cells, each of which produces millions of antibodies. These antibodies then head for the antigens using the bloodstream. Large numbers lock onto the antigens and disable it. They are assisted by what is called complement. It acts as a catalyst for the reaction between the antibodies and the antigen, and it speed up the reaction. It helps neutralize viruses and other unfriendly microbes.

Phagocytes

Two other types of cells are also important in the fight against antigens. They are the neutrophils and macrophages. Known as phagocytes, they attack and eat antigens. Both are born in bone marrow, and they mature relatively fast. Neurophils are much smaller than macrophages. They are like foot soldiers - lightly armed, but there are large numbers of them, and they are usually the first to attack the antigens. When called into battle they rush in, but can only kill and eat a few antigens (10 to 20) before they die.

Macrophages start out in the thymus as monophages. When they migrate to lymphatic tissue they grow by a factor of 4 or 5 and become macrophages. They are much larger and better trained than neutrophils and they can engulf and eat up to 100 antigens. One of their major jobs is to cut microbes up into small pieces, each displaying their antigen, signaling that they are the enemy.

Summary of the Fight Between the Immune System and Foreign Antigens

The events that occur when your body has been attacked are quite complex and complicated, but I'll give a simple version of it.

1. A virus of other pathogen invades you body. It gains entry through your nose, eyes, mouth or perhaps a cut.
2. Nearby macrophages and helper T cells usually detect it first. They head for the site of infection.

3. Macrophages cut up the source so that the antigens can be checked to see if they are friend or enemy.

4. Many T-4's arrive at the site. They release cytokines that alert all parts of the immune system.

5. The T-4 cells proliferate, producing other helper cells, suppressors, and killer cells. All recognize the particular antigen.

6. Some of the T-4's go to the lymph nodes where they release messengers to alert the B-cells and authorize them to produce antibodies.

7. The B-cells change into plasma cells and each plasma cell produces millions of antibodies. All of this takes time, however, depending on the health of your system. A typical time is a few days, but it may be much longer if your immune system is weak.

8. In the meantime the virus, or pathogens, are producing thousands of copies of themselves and they are fighting back to avoid detection and death.

9. The NK and killer T-cells begin attacking the viruses. But hundreds of thousands of viruses have been produced and the lymphocytes are overwhelmed at first. Some of the viruses are now migrating to other parts of the body.

10. The immune system increases the temperature

of the body in an effort to destroy the invaders. It may increase it to 104 degrees. It also sends in inflammation to wall off the invaders in an effort to stop them from spreading.

11. After several days the antibodies and complement begin to make some progress. Finally the antibodies, complement, NK and killer T's along with neutrophils and macrophages begin fighting in unison and begin to overcome the invaders.

12. The immune system is now very aggressive, however, and must be turned off when the battle is over. This is where the T-8's come in.

It's easy to see from this why you need a strong and healthy immune system. Delays at any stage after the infection allows the antigens to multiply and if not stopped they can overcome your body.

Chain Reaction of Bad Health Possible Without Help

Your immune system is very important to your health. A strong immune system can prevent you from developing many diseases. When your immune system is compromised you become more susceptible to illness. There are many ways you may be harming your immunity. You can follow many simple guidelines to keep your immunity in top shape.

Food Choices: The foods you choose to eat can have a

tremendous impact on your immune system. There are several types of food that you should avoid or definitely limit your consumption of. Sugar: Eating too much sugar can spike insulin levels. It also can affect your body's ability to absorb nutrients, particularly vitamin C. Eat sugary snacks in moderation or special occasions. Stevia is a wonderful, natural sugar that you can use in place of regular sugar. Protein: We need protein for our health. You should eat lean proteins such as chicken, turkey and fish. Avoid fatty beef and pork. If you do consume them eat the white meat pork and leaner cuts of beef. Too much protein will be stored as fat in the body. Over time this can weaken your immunity.

Poor Nutrition: Many people live a fast paced lifestyle and eat their food on the run throughout the day. Often grabbing fast food for breakfast and lunch, this way of eating will not give your body the complete nutrition that it requires for optimal health. Take the time to plan out your meals for the week. You can learn to make quick and nutritious meals and avoid the fast food trap. For example, a simple and easy breakfast can be a plain yogurt with fruit and granola. Lunch can be a premade salad with lean protein such as turkey or chicken added in. Easy snacks to carry with you include nuts and fresh and dried fruit. Dinner can be a simple and easy to make grilled fish with sautéed vegetables. You will begin to feel healthier if you incorporate more nutrition in your diet. Fast food and processed products will wreak havoc on your health if you continue on this path for too long. It will rob you of your energy and cause weight gain.

Bad Fats: There are good and bad fats. Good fats that you want to eat are Omega-3 fatty acids. These can be found in fresh seafood such as tuna and salmon. Enjoy olive oil on your vegetables, salads and rice dishes as this oil is also very healthy to consume. You want to avoid the bad fats which include those found in fatty cuts of beef and pork. Too much bad fat can potentially lead to toxic buildup in the body, including the digestive system and weaken your immunity. Alcohol: Limit your alcohol consumption. Excess alcohol consumption can lead to a weaker immune system as it can suppress white blood cells. Smoking: This goes without saying; smoking will wreak havoc on your health and your immunity. If you are a smoker you should see your medical doctor. He or she will be able to assist you in finding ways to quit this unhealthy habit. Water: You need plenty of fresh clean water on a daily basis. Most people do not drink enough water. Water helps flush your body of toxins helping your immune system to not have to work as hard. Try to limit your intake of sugary soda and fruit juices high in sugar.

Sleep: Getting enough sleep nightly can have a big

impact on your overall health. When you sleep your body is in a process of regenerating. When you do not get enough sleep your body cannot repair itself properly and therefore your immune system may suffer. Stress: Stress has deleterious effects on the human body. Continued prolonged stress will deplete your energy and harm your immunity. We must all deal with stress but it is important to incorporate healthy lifestyle choices to reduce your stress levels as much as possible. Lack of exercise: Being sedentary can also weaken immunity. The human body is meant to be physically active. Moderate, consistent exercise is very healthy. You need to find exercise activities that interest you and that you can make a reasonable commitment to stick with.

Aging and Immunity: As we age our bodies naturally decline and of course this includes the immune system. You need to strive to lead as healthy of a lifestyle as you can to compensate for this natural aging process. Aging can also lead to a higher probability of injuries to areas like the knees and hips. If you injure yourself you place stress on your immune system. This is where a good exercise program can help to keep you limber and strong as you age. Remember whenever beginning any dietary or lifestyle changes, always consult with a medical professional, particularly if you are taking prescription drugs or suffer from any disease or ailment.

If you don't get the help you need for your immune system you might find that your body is in serious need of assistance. Unfortunately, most people don't realize there is a problem with their natural immunity until it has become a really big problem. The fact remains that big problems with this system can prove deadly if left unchecked.

CHAPTER 8

THE IMPORTANT ROLE OF NUTRITION ON IMMUNITY

Whenever we take any food or nourishing liquids, our body digests and absorbs the simple but essential minerals, vitamins, fats, proteins, carbohydrates, fats and water from these foods or nourishing liquids and converts it into the bloodstream and energy that help our body to grow and keep it healthy.

The nutrition value is more important for any individual's health. The food or liquids whenever we take it affect our body and health as well both. So it is very important that we should be more aware of the foods or liquids whatever we take in our daily life. A large number of diseases occur only due to wrong diet. Some certain diet may itself cause some disease or alter the course of a known disorder such as diabetes, heart or kidney disease.

As we know that food and water is necessary to build up our body and keep it healthy. Every good food and liquid contains some important nutrition like proteins, carbohydrate, fats, some vitamins, minerals and water. These all play different role to keep our body healthy and build new cells in our body.

One of the best things to do to boost immunity is eat foods that are designed for that purpose in large amounts. Unfortunately, not everyone is interested in 30 or so servings of broccoli each week. The result is that most people do not get the proper nutrition to keep their immune systems in good working order. For those people other action needs to be taken.

Sleep Deprivation and Immunity

If you're not consistently getting adequate sleep then it's probably taking a toll on your overall health and sense of well-being. It may surprise you to learn that chronic sleep deprivation significantly affects your immune system, alertness at work, memory, safety, and pocketbook.

The following are some of the consequences of sleep deprivation:

Reduced Energy, Performance, and Alertness on the Job: Reducing your rejuvenating sleep by as little as one and a half hours for just one night could result in a decrease of daytime alertness by as much as 32%.

Memory and Cognitive Impairment: Decreased

alertness and excessive daytime sleepiness negatively affects your memory and your ability to efficiently think and process information.

Stress in Relationships: Disruption of a bed partner's sleep due to a sleep disorder may cause problems in relationships (sleeping separate bedrooms, conflicts, moodiness, etc.).

Poor Quality of Life: You may be unable to participate in certain activities that require sustained attention, like going to the movies, seeing your child in a school play, or watching a favorite TV show.

Occupational Hazard: Sleep deprivation also contributes to a greater than twofold higher risk of sustaining an occupational injury.

Automobile Injury: The National Highway Traffic Safety Administration (NHTSA) estimates conservatively that each year drowsy driving is responsible for at least 100,000 automobile crashes, 71,000 injuries, and 1,550 fatalities.

The human body's sleep cycles are intricately connected to the earth in what is known as circadian rhythms. Yawning is due to lack of oxygen. This is why we get tired. Exhaustion and fatigue is due to lack of oxygen in the body. Lack of oxygen over time results in the body being more acidic. The body rejuvenates itself more speedily during nighttime sleep so the more restful your sleep, the better chance you have of achieving perfect wellness.

Rapid eye movement sleep in adult humans typically occupies 20-25% of total sleep, about 90-120 minutes of a night's sleep. During an average night of sleep, you should experience about four or five periods of REM sleep; they are quite brief at the beginning of the night and longer toward the end. The need for REM sleep decreases with age. A typical newborn will spend about 80% of sleep time in Rapid eye movement sleep.

Dream-deprived sleep after three nights means you'll soon be in a psychiatric ward. It has a seriously adverse effects on the brain's normal function. Drug addicts and alcoholics don't dream very much because the excessive "brain-altering" substance prevents the brain from experiencing these natural phases. The Rapid eye movement phases are necessary for your brain function. If you overload your short-term memory, you will "get crazy." The short-term memory goes through a filtering process during the REM cycle and as a result, memories which are relevant are further strengthened, while weaker, transient, "noise" memories will get dumped. This is your Intelligent Body at work.

Eight hours of sleep is ideal but most people can get by on six or seven. Any less than five and you may be interfering with the Rapid eye movement phases. To be more in tune with the earth and its circadian rhythms, I suggest going to bed as early as possible after sundown. The more sleep you get closer to dusk, the better chance you'll have of completing your Rapid eye movement periods and getting a deep, replenishing, and restful sleep.

If you want to wear a body down go for a while with too little sleep. It's great to work and play hard but you need to understand the toll that these things take on your body. If you plan to keep long hours or burn your candle at both ends and the middle, then you need help so that you can keep going at the pace you must manage. Most people, though aren't interested in sacrificing their lifestyles for the sake of a stronger immune system if there are options available.

CHAPTER 9

TURNING TO HYPNOSIS
FOR HELP

In our society, we are bombarded by fast paced changes and many daily challenges. As a result, our lives are full of stresses in our personal life and relationships, our careers, job settings and the demands on our time. In addition, the current economic climate creates additional stresses such as those stresses related to being unemployed and being able to meet financial obligations to keep a home and paying for food, utilities.

It has long been known there is a direct relationship between people experiencing long-term stress, developing illnesses and having long recovery times from simple colds or injuries and worse. Those who have learned to manage their stress levels are less prone to stress related illness and are able to recover much quicker. So, learning to manage your stress levels will affect how well your immune system keeps you healthy.

Hypnosis is an exceedingly effective method for managing emotional issues such as anxiety, fear and physical and mental stress. Hypnosis helps to relax your mind and body by reducing the effects of the emotional stressors and allowing your mind and body to reset your stress levels to a more manageable state day to day.

Help might very well be as simple as self-hypnosis. Hypnosis can send the signals your body needs to work more efficiently leaving left over nutrients available to the immune system. Hypnosis can also be used to keep you stress free and warding off the illnesses that nick away at the potency of your immune system day after day.

One of the most popular and successful psychological methods for the treatment of physical illness is hypnosis. How the hypnotic process actually works is, surprisingly, still a mystery to modern science. However, its effects are well documented.

Although many people consider hypnosis to be some form of mind control that is influenced upon you by another person this could not be further from the truth. Because we give the hypnotist permission to guide us into trance all hypnosis is actually self-hypnosis. You do not surrender your will to a hypnotist nor would you follow his every instruction blindly.

When you are hypnotized you are still in full control. However, as you have agreed to surrender a certain amount of control to the hypnotist you feel that you want to please him and are much more likely to accept his suggestions and believe everything he says.

So, how can this self-hypnosis state be used to promote better states of physical well-being and even eliminate some illnesses?

Well, research has shown that our thoughts have a dramatic effect on our health and general well-being. Our thoughts themselves are merely reflections of the believe we hold and these beliefs are themselves slaves to our emotions. Our emotions, in turn, are greatly influenced by our past experiences and how we view them in the present. Being able to alter all of these is one of the most powerful benefits of using self-hypnosis.

Through self-hypnosis it is possible to alter how we view our past experiences and remove or change the emotional charges we hold against them. Similarly we can also create visions of our future, with self-hypnosis, and infuse these visualizations with positive, affirming emotions. The visions produced under self-hypnosis are stored in the mind for latter access. When the mind calls up information from its subconscious storehouse it then reads from these visions and uses them as a blueprint for how it views the world.

As a health-aid it is therefore the role of self-hypnosis to alter our internal belief systems to correspond to thinking process that promote health and general good well-being. To achieve this our emotions to certain beliefs must also be changed. This has proven to be difficult, time-consuming and slow with conventional psychological methods - this is not the case with self-hypnosis however!

Anyone can use self-hypnosis to enter a state of trance. Once in this relaxed state worded statements can be directed to the subconscious mind and visualization techniques used to change beliefs, thoughts, emotions and behaviors. This can be achieved with any subject matter. In fact, it can take as little as one session to accomplish this and no more than a few sessions a week over a period of one month.

As far as health goes self-hypnosis can create dramatic changes in the body. As the human brain is the center, or controller, of the complex nervous system of the body it has the ability to send and receive signals from all parts of the body. The brain's ability to be in contact with the whole body and send instructions means that it has the ability to instruct cells and nerves to begin repair or reconstruction of any damaged system. As you can have direct access to the brain you can literally program it with your own instructions!

With self-hypnosis you can gain access to the part of the mind known as the subconscious and program in instructions that have a dramatic effect on how the brain interacts with the nerves and cells of your body. Through the use of self-hypnosis techniques you can actually change the blueprint your mind holds of your body to reflect health, strength and wellness. When the brain then accesses the subconscious mind to send instructions to your nerves and cells it reads this newly programmed blueprint imprinted on it through self-hypnosis and immediately instructs the rest of the body to follow it - much like a computer system.

Therefore if your health is an issue that you would like to deal with my advice is simple. Apply some easy to learn self-hypnosis techniques or use well-established self-hypnosis recordings and you will change your mind and ultimately your body!

Are you ready to enjoy a steady diet of broccoli and other immunity boosting vegetables at every meal in your day? Do you want to give up late night activities so that you can go to bed early each night ensuring adequate rest? Or are you ready to give self-hypnosis for immune system help a try today?

CHAPTER 10

WHAT DOES NUTRITION HAVE TO DO WITH IMMUNE SYSTEM

The immune system is a "complex network of specialized organs, cells, and substances". It includes the skin, stomach, pancreas, bone marrow, spleen, liver, thymus gland, tonsils, and the lymphatic system- basically, "all cells and tissues of the body that have the ability to resist infection and disease." There are patches of lymphoid tissue in the intestinal tract, as well.

"Immunity is the ability of the body to defend itself against specific invading agents such as bacteria, toxins, viruses, and foreign tissues." Immunity provides a mechanism for defense against disease. Immunity on a cellular level is what protects us against fungi, viruses, bacteria and yeast infections. For example, "B-Cells, T-Cells and antibodies protect all body systems from attack by harmful foreign invaders (pathogens), foreign cells, and cancer cells."

Nutrition plays a significant role in a healthy immune

system. Considering that the immune system is a multi-organ system, and that there are millions of new immune system cells are produced daily, it is reasonable to assume that "its large size and high cellular turnover combine to make the immune system a major consumer of nutrients. So, some aspects of immunity are very sensitive to nutritional deficiencies. It is uncertain as to whether this decline in immunity results from nutritional deficiencies and/or increased requirements. The latter could result from a variety of causes which will be discussed later. Human studies have shown that there is a "causal association between under-nutrition and secondary immune-depression that results in diminished resistance to infectious diseases" and that "severe malnutrition has a major impact on resistance to disease that is partly mediated through the immune system. There is also evidence that "moderate-to-marginal under-nutrition may compromise immunity". Deficiencies of zinc, folic acid, essential fatty acids, manganese, calcium or any one of the B vitamins may severe impair immune system functioning. "Studies confirm that becoming depleted in even one nutrient can cause us to suffer a variety of ailments and can certainly predispose us to inflation, allergies, and even cancer".

New research has shown that a deficiency in one or more of 8 essential monosaccharides can impair immunity as they "combine with proteins and fats on cell surfaces to influence cell-to-cell communication and the functioning of the immune system.

Natural medicine sees the value of preventing disease, in comparison to reacting to it. There are certain foods have been shown to strengthen the immune system. Plums, broccoli and other green leafy vegetables, sea veggies, mushrooms, and aloe vera are "power foods"- foods that offer special benefits in relation to immune system support.

Plums, either fresh or dried, have been the subject of repeated health research because of their high content of unique phytonutrients, classified as phenols and their function as antioxidants has been well-documented. Plums increase absorption of iron into the body which has been documented in published research and this ability may be due the high content of vitamin C in this fruit. In addition, to assisting with absorption of iron, vitamin C is needed in the body to make healthy tissue and is also needed for a strong immune system. Plums are a good source of vitamin A (in the form of beta-carotene), vitamin B2, dietary fiber and potassium and come in over 2,000 varieties.

Broccoli, and other cruciferous vegetables like brussel sprouts, are excellent sources of vitamin A (beta-carotene), B, C and E, incomplete proteins and calcium and are high in fiber. The phytonutrients in broccoli along with our own enzymes optimize our cells' ability to disarm and clear free radicals and toxins, including potential carcinogens. Recent studies show that those eating the most cruciferous vegetables have a much lower risk of prostate, colorectal and lung cancer-even when compared to those who regularly eat other vegetables. For example, in 1992 "a researcher at John Hopkins University announced the discovery of a compound found in broccoli, namely polyphenols, that not only prevented the development of tumors by 60% in the studied group, it also reduced the size of tumors that did develop by 75%. In a study of over 1,000 men conducted at the Fred Hutchinson Cancer Research Center in Seattle, WA, those eating 28 servings of vegetables a week had a 35% lower risk of prostate cancer, but those consuming just 3 or more servings of cruciferous vegetables each week had a 44% lower prostate cancer risk.

In the Netherlands Cohort Study on Diet and Cancer, in which data was collected on over 100,000 people for more than 6 years, those eating the most vegetables benefited with a 25% lower risk of colorectal cancers, but those eating the most cruciferous vegetables did almost twice as well with a 49% drop in their colorectal cancer risk. A study of Chinese women in Singapore, a city in which air pollution levels are often high putting stress on the detoxification capacity of residents' lungs, found that in non-smokers, eating cruciferous vegetables lowered risk of lung cancer by 30%. In smokers, regular cruciferous vegetable consumption reduced lung cancer risk an amazing 69%. One cup of broccoli contains the RDA for vitamin C, and fortifies the immune system with beta-carotene, and small but useful amounts of zinc and selenium, two trace minerals that act as cofactors in numerous immune defensive actions.

A combination of these and other power foods have the ability to defend, protect and restore. They act to defend the immune system by enhancing cell-to-cell communication, allowing the cells to send and receive messages clearly and effectively. They protect against the various environmental toxins, poor food sources, and stress. Power foods help to restore cellular health that has been compromised by pollutants; such as those in the air we breathe and water we drink.

Sea vegetables, more commonly known as seaweed or marine algae, have superior nutritional value that enhances immune system function. Wakame, undaria pinnatifida, is one of the most important species of seaweed that is rich in protein, calcium, iodine, magnesium, iron and folate. Lignans, which help fight cancer are found in high quantity in wakame (kelp) and may provide protection against certain cancers.

Spirulina is a spiral-shaped, blue-green, single-celled alga. It is an over 65% complete, pre-digested vegetable protein. Spirulina absorbs and retains many minerals and nutrients including essential fatty acids, GLA fatty acid, lipids, the nucleic acids (RNA and DNA), B complex, vitamin C and E, and phytochemicals such as carotenoids, chlorophyll (blood purifier) and phycocyanin, a protein that is known to inhibit cancer.

Shitake, reishi and mitake mushrooms contribute to increased cellular immunity and have been shown to promote the conversion of cancer cells to normal cells. Chinese research supports the use of these mushrooms to stimulate immune function. They contain betaglucans that are proven immunostimulants. Mushrooms have good nutritional value because they are low in calories and fat and have no cholesterol. They are low in salt and contain various minerals including potassium, linoleic acid, folate, copper, iron, phosphorus, magnesium and selenium. Mushrooms include a good source of vitamins especially B vitamins. The protein found in mushrooms is superior to other vegetable protein due its essential amino acid content. Between 70-90% of this vegetable protein can be easily digested.

Aloe Vera, a common plant, has been used for thousands of years on burns and cuts. More significantly, it includes an abundance of essential sugars needed for cellular communication. Aloe appears to strengthen the immune system, particularly in those already healthy, to keep patient from contracting other infections. It has a high antioxidant capacity and an anti-inflammatory effect.

The following dietary guidelines are contributing factors in enhancing immune system functioning:

1) limit the intake of white sugar and refined flour products;
2) drink plenty of water;
3) use whole grains;
4) limit the intake of fatty dairy products, and;
5) increase the consumption of fresh fruits, vegetables and legumes.

The Organic Trade Association has cited several reasons to eat organic foods. Some of the most important reasons, in my estimation include the fact that organic products meet stringent standards-reducing health risks by eliminating the use of toxic chemicals, and that organic farmers build healthy soils- the foundation of the food chain. Healthier soils will promote higher nutritive value in foods.

Eating a combination of raw and cooked foods may provide maximum health benefits. For example, raw and cooked broccoli (crucifers) provides different anticancer phytonutrients. The raw vegetable has higher vitamin C but cooking the vegetable makes the carotenoids more bioavailable.

CHAPTER 11

EATING RIGHT FOR
A HEALTHY IMMUNE SYSTEM

Experts in the medical science field once worried about influenza. Today the focus seems to have turned to 'afflulenza'. Lifestyle diseases, more than anything else, are snuffing out lives and shortening productive years of the population. Leading the way for immune system disorders.

The mind-set today seems to be to get rich, buy cars, get houses and get meals out. I see it every day. Husband and wife both working, and working longer hours to pay the bills. When we chase such a lifestyle what we get in return is appalling. We get obesity, cardiovascular diseases, diabetes, respiratory problems and cancer. Despite the progress in medical science, there are sure cures for a very small number of ailments.

Besides that, there is an extraordinary level of reliance on the antibiotic alternative as patients and doctors are in a hurry to earn the next buck, which does not make things any better. Herbal antibiotics, on the other hand, treats ailments and boosts the functions of the immune system.

Besides the visible physical problems, a prolonged illness can wreck mental health and can also negatively affect a healthy immune system. It can hinder the body's capacities to self-heal. Immune system is a relatively new area of study for the medical experts and not much is known about the mechanisms of its dysfunction.

However, it has been established that certain factors that there are certain factors that affect immune system health. The way we eat and what we eat is one of them.

The immune system, which is primarily responsible for recognizing foreign substances like bacteria and toxins must be in proper shape to perform its function of destroying such foreign material. A weakened immune system is a cause to disease in two ways.

It is unable of fighting infections and you are therefore susceptible to contracting diseases more often. The immune system also looses its capability to recognize foreign invasions and starts destroying the body's own normal cells, which causes autoimmune diseases like rheumatoid arthritis and diabetes.

Food has been the first of all casualties behind the

gradual decline of traditional family patterns and eating practices. We may be eating more calories but we are obtaining them from poor sources, eating fat of inferior quality (trans-fats), more sugar, refined carbohydrates, more meat, chemicals and preservatives. This type of diet can adversely affect the body's self-healing capacity.

Instead of the vitamins to boost your immune system and dietary supplements that you may choose to add on to your food, opt to eat certain foods that help your immune system. Vitamin C in combination with magnesium and calcium resists infections. For people who have problems of heartburn, citrus fruits may not be advisable as they are highly acidic in nature.

Crab meat, lobsters and oysters are rich in all three nutrients - calcium, magnesium and Vitamin C. Salmon is rich in a lot of minerals and vitamins along with a substantial quantity of Omega 3 fatty acids. Omega 3 fatty acids are good for arthritis and heart disease and also aid immune system functioning. Other healthy sources of Vitamin C are broccoli, tomatoes, peaches and guava.

Selenium is a trace mineral that is essential for immune system health, which you will not find in multi-vitamin supplements. Chicken and broccoli are healthy sources of selenium. Different types of edible mushrooms increase the production of white blood cells, which are essential for effectively combating disease.

A case also exists for the use of herbs for immune system. These are herbs that our ancestors used, to maintain health and vitality. These herbs are still an integral part of traditional therapies and the mainstay of homoeopathy.

Foods That Boost the Immune System

Recommendations for foods that boost the immune system vary. The Chinese diet to boost the immune system includes a chicken soup tonic that contains chicken, deng shen, broomrape, and sliced ginger. Prevention magazine recommends beef, sweet potatoes, mushrooms, tea and yogurt. Other experts recommend avoiding beef and eating a diet rich in vegetables like broccoli, cabbage, Brussels sprouts and cauliflower, because of the enzymes they contain. Any or all of these diets could have merit. The primary goal should be overall good nutrition.

There are a number of vitamins, minerals, plant components and herbs that are beneficial to the immune system. Finding specific foods that boost the immune system can be complicated, because certain vitamins work best when taken with other vitamins. For instance, vitamin C, probably the most commonly recommended vitamin for infection resistance, works best when taken with calcium and magnesium. Calcium, among the other vital roles that it plays in the body, helps the cells absorb Vitamin C and other nutrients more efficiently. Magnesium plays the same role and is also essential for proper function of the muscles and nerves. So, an effective diet to boost the immune system must include foods that contain Vitamin C, magnesium and calcium, or a combination of foods that contain these important nutrients.

To further complicate your search for foods that boost the immune system, calcium and magnesium, which are necessary for the proper absorption of Vitamin C, work best when taken with iron, manganese, and Vitamin D. The body cannot absorb calcium, if Vitamin D is not present, which is why milk is fortified with Vitamin D. In addition, a lack of Vitamin A in the diet can lead to frequent infections and Vitamin A works best when taken with zinc, calcium, B-complex, and vitamins C, D and E. You may at this point give up on a diet to boost the immune system and just take a multi-vitamin instead, but not all multi-vitamins are the same. Some do not contain calcium or iron. Some are properly balanced for men, but not for women.

Even if you take a good daily multi-vitamin, it is still important to eat a healthy diet and there are some interesting foods that boost the immune system, according to recent studies. Edible mushrooms, for example, are a valuable source of biologically active compounds called beta glucans and could benefit a diet to boost the immune system. Numerous studies have shown that beta glucans stimulate the immune system, providing protection from colds, influenza and infections, as well as AIDS by inhibiting viral replication. If you prefer not to eat mushrooms, beta glucans are found in numerous plant foods, including oats, barley and yeast.

Crabmeat, lobster, oysters, salmon and tuna are all foods that boost the immune system. Because, they are good sources of calcium, magnesium, manganese, iron and vitamins A, C, D, E and B complex. Dieticians and nutritionists often refer to salmon as a "super food". It not only contains all of the vitamins and minerals necessary to maintain a healthy immune system, but is also rich in Omega-3 fatty acids, which are believed to be beneficial in preventing heart disease, cancer and arthritis. Omega-3 supplementation can improve overall mental function and reduce symptoms of depression. Dietary experts recommend two servings of salmon per week or four servings of tuna, not only to be included in a diet to boost the immune system, but also to provide adequate amounts of omega-3 fatty acids.

Certainly, there is no specific diet to boost the immune system, but eating a well-balanced diet will improve immune system function. There are foods that boost the immune system because of the vitamins and minerals that they contain, but of utmost importance is overall good nutrition. The best protection is obtained by eating the right foods in the right combination whenever possible, supplementing with a daily multi-vitamin and possibly a natural immune system enhancer during cold and flu season or whenever you feel you are at risk for infection.

Journey To Healing and Health

We often say: my heart's not in it anymore; my heart is sore; my heart is breaking. This is much more literal than we thought! In all cultures and religions, the experience of peace, love, healing and harmony are seated in the heart and thymus (responsible for immunity) region in the chest. Feelings of love also have a positive influence on the immune system, hormones and cognitive brain function.

Healing ideas for your heart

Opening your heart to healing your physical body to release cell memories, optimise physical health and use the body to connect you to your mind, emotions and soul essence

Identify body signals of severe stress: feel the pain, anxiety, restlessness, insomnia, depression.

Breathing exercises to open the chest area, expand the

lungs, increase oxygenation of cells: belly or diaphragmatic breathing, bellows breathing, alternate nostril breathing.

Progressive deep muscle relaxation.

Specific yoga exercises: head, neck and shoulder stretches and rotations; cobra pose; half locust pose; head-to-knee pose; forward bending pose; shoulder stand, even if you simply lift your feet onto the seat of a chair; chest extension or fish pose; spinal twist; sun salutation; dead man's pose to end.

Work with arms - reaching out, drawing in with dance movements such as Nia technique, and slow, mindful movement like Tai 'chi.

Following a heart health eating plan.

Using heart health food supplements and herbal remedies.

Opening your heart to healing your emotions or feelings towards yourself and others

Work on releasing past emotional injuries and hurts.

Forgiveness of self and others.

Work on relationships, release of sorrow, guilt, acceptance of self and others.

Anger management: learn how to acknowledge the intense energy of anger and allow it proper expression.

Opening your heart to healing your thoughts use heart centered positive affirmations and directed visualizations to sense feelings of love, joy, peace and happiness within the heart. Also using the image of the sun, placing it in the heart and then allowing the moon to place itself over the heart. This allows for a balance of male and female energies within the heart.

Go on a journey of self-discovery: deeply ingrained unconscious patterns of behavior that do not serve you any longer, through journaling, psychotherapy, free hand writing

Opening your heart to connect to your soul, meditate regularly. mindfulness, witnessing, visualization meditations work well for the heart. Releasing the shadow deep inside the unconscious mind through transpersonal and soul based psychotherapy. Quiet time, soul reflection and contemplation.

CHAPTER 12

HEALING FROM WITHIN OUR IMMUNE SYSTEM

In our technologically advanced society, why have the advocates of traditional medicine not found a cure for the common cold?

The reason is that the common cold is not the problem; it is only the effect or symptom of the underlying problem.

And why have the practitioners and researchers of traditional medicine failed to realize that?

The reason is that the supporters of traditional medicine still maintain that the universe is material at its core; and therefore they continue to treat the symptoms rather than the invisible causes because the symptoms are material and palpable. And they continue to do so 81 years after physicists discovered in 1925 that atoms were made out of energy. So if energy makes atoms, and atoms make molecules, and molecules make cells, and cells make us, then we, too, are energy.

The supporters of traditional medicine have also been wrong about what causes stress. Stress is not caused by our external environment; stress is caused by what we perceive our external environment to be. For example, darkness may cause stress in one person; whereas it has no effect on another person.

Our autonomic nervous systems are our bodies' control center for stress. Our autonomic nervous systems are divided into the parasympathetic nervous systems and the sympathetic nervous systems.

Our parasympathetic nervous systems control our bodies' involuntary functions such as our immune systems, digestive systems, cardiovascular systems, neurological systems, and reproductive systems. During this normal body functioning, our cells are in a growth mode and our bodies' immune systems are healing our bodies.

Our sympathetic nervous systems are activated when we perceive danger, whether real or imagined; and that perception of danger causes our stress. As our bodies ready themselves for immediate physical activity, they are now in a fight or flight mode. Our sympathetic nervous systems send adrenalin, glucose, and oxygen to our organs most active in warding off danger. Our cells now shift from a growth mode to a self-protection mode. And when our cells are in a self-protection mode, our immune systems shut down and are no longer available to heal our bodies. But when stress disappears, our autonomic nervous systems automatically shift our cells back into growth mode; and our immune systems are available again to heal our bodies. Our bodies are now in homeostasis or normal body functioning.

But what happens if stress remains in our bodies? If stress remains in our bodies, whether or not we are conscious of it, our cells remain in a self-protection mode, and illness, disease, and disorder manifests.

So how do we eradicate stress from our bodies? How do we return our cells to growth mode? How do we activate our immune systems to again heal and protect our bodies?

It was Hippocrates who once said, "A wise man should consider that health is the greatest of human blessings". He was so right when he said that, and we only really agree with that once illness strike. Many of us cannot even cope with a common cold. We run to the doctor with our first sneeze. We do not even try to fight the cold ourselves. The reason I believe, is a lack of knowledge of the inner power of healing.

Nature has provided us with an amazing immune system that has the power to combat any illness or disease, provided we take good care of our immune system. The problem is our modern lifestyle has caused us to be ignorant towards our immune system.

We eat junk food, we abuse alcohol, we are dependent on all kinds of drugs and we live in a polluted environment coupled with all the stress in the world. Even though we live in an age where all the information in the world is freely available to everybody, we choose to be ignorant towards it. We choose to live the fast and instant life. Most of us have a profound lack of knowledge as to what our bodies need to function optimally and thus we find ourselves susceptible to all sorts of illnesses.

Nature has intended to provide us with all the right natural substances to fuel our immune systems and enable our bodies to function up to its fullest potential. The resources nature provides are whole foods, vitamins and minerals, enzymes and amino acids and phytochemicals. It is up to every individual to take up the responsibility of the maintenance of their health and in the treatment of disorders. Each person has the responsibility and ability to learn about nutrition and nurturing the immune system. Prevention is always better than cure, and if we take care of our inner healing power, our immune systems, then many of the chronic lifestyle diseases will not even touch us.

The human body is a very complex organism that has been given the ability to heal itself. We must listen to our bodies and respond with the right nourishment and care. Many of us have for many years abused our own bodies through smoking, abusing alcohol, unhealthy eating and lack of exercise. Even with all those abuse our bodies still serve us well for many years while crying out for better treatment. If we do not respond, then all of a sudden illnesses start to appear. But it is still not too late. If within the onset of illness, we would respond and nourish our immune systems, healing can start from within and years can be added to our lives.

CHAPTER 13

HOW TO RESTORE
OVERALL HEALTH

Optimum nutrition is considered to be a revolution in health care. When you fuel your body with optimum nutrition, you are giving yourself the best possible intake of nutrients to enable your body to function and be as healthy as possible. The nutrition is what helps your body perform all sorts of basic functions...detoxification, strengthens your immune system, provides natural antioxidants, and provides digestive enzymes...to name a few.

Preventing or reversing disease-states is but one more function of optimum nutrition. Science is showing us every day that nutritional deficiency is contributing largely, if not actually causing, illness and disease in our bodies. But optimum nutrition is about more than just keeping disease and illness at bay. It is about living optimally, where we have room to stretch our physical, mental, and spiritual "muscles" to the full, without overstepping the threshold at which cellular health in any of the systems of the body becomes threatened.

Your nutritional goal should be to give yourself the best possible intake of nutrients to enable your body to function and be as healthy as possible. Optimum nutrition consists of eating the right amounts of nutrients on a proper schedule to achieve the best performance and the longest possible lifetime in good health. When you are providing the proper balance of nutrients to your body, your daily diet will consist of the right quantities of protein, fat, carbohydrates, vitamins, minerals, and fiber to maintain a healthy body and to sustain the desired level of activity for the best quality of life.

Apart from being essential to general good health, optimum nutrition is so fundamental and powerful that it can speed healing and improve weight, energy, immune functions, sleep, mental acuity, feelings, attitude and just about any aspect of your being. It is a state of profound physical, mental and emotional well-being. Optimum nutrition is within all of our grasps; it starts with a commitment to a lifestyle.

HEALTH

How do you define health? Is it a state of complete physical, mental and social well-being? Is it merely the absence of disease or infirmity? Or is health a resource for everyday life, rather than the objective of living; a positive concept, emphasizing social and personal resources as well as physical capabilities?

Good health is harder to define than bad health (which can be equated with the presence of disease), because it must convey a concept more positive than mere absence of disease, and there is a variable area between health and disease. Health is clearly a complex, multidimensional concept. Health is, ultimately, poorly defined and difficult to measure, despite impressive efforts by epidemiologists, vital statisticians, social scientists and political economists. Each individual's health is shaped by many factors, including medical care, social circumstances, and behavioral choices.

Health is not merely the absence of pain or tension, but it is a joy in living; a real appreciation of what it is to have a healthy body with which to experience the many pleasures of this world. While it may sound simple...this isn't an easy task.

Because of the nature of processed food and depleted soils, most nutritional experts believe that the current diet provides enough vitamins and minerals for survival, but not for optimal health. Minimizing the intake of processed foods is essential for restoring your digestive health.

Many health benefits are due to another group of health-promoting nutrients called phytochemicals, which are found in fresh, raw fruits and vegetables. Now, that's coming back to the basics. Yet many people continue to be surprised that something as simple as coming back to basic nutrition, balancing your diet, and keeping healthy can go a long way to relieving daily aggravations such as skin problems, slowing down signs of aging, and keeping you looking better year after year.

Personal or individual health is largely subjective. For most individuals and for many cultures, however, health is a philosophical and subjective concept, associated with contentment, and often taken for granted when all is going well. The evidence that behavioral factors such as diet, physical activity, smoking and stress influence health is overwhelming. Thus, health is maintained and improved not only through the advancement and application of health science, but also through the efforts and intelligent lifestyle choices of the individual and society. Perhaps the best thing you can do for your health is to keep a positive attitude. Optimal health can be defined as a balance of physical, emotional, social, spiritual and intellectual health. Maintain a positive attitude!

QUALITY

So, the fact is that food is not only vital fuel, but also fundamental "medicine"...and it is vital that we pay attention to the quality and quantity of fuel that we feed our bodies. Optimum nutrition helps the body to cleanse and repair itself, restore energy levels, rebalance hormones, the blood sugar level, brain chemicals, and generally improve one's quality of life. The quality and balance of our food intake is therefore a key factor in determining our overall health.

In whole foods, you will find the greatest concentration of quality nutrition per calorie of intake. Research has shown that optimum nutrition is achieved through the eating of a variety of natural foods that are packed with vitamins and minerals. It is about finding the foods and nutrients that will help you achieve better health and vitality, and avoiding those that may not suit you. Once optimum nutrition is in place, you can look forward to a consistent high level of energy, emotional balance, alertness, physical fitness, resilience against infectious diseases, and longevity.

Improving your overall health starts with being health conscious, making smart lifestyle choices and focusing on preventative care. Today's fast-paced economy has created a mindset of instant gratification even when health is involved. People want to take a pill and instantly feel a difference, and many do not see value in preventative therapies unless they see a problem first. With poor lifestyle choices today consisting of fad diets, eating processed foods, taking prescription medication, consuming alcohol, over indulging in sweets and artificial sweeteners, the body is working in overdrive to rid itself of toxins and reduce body-wide inflammation. If more time was spent focusing on natural alternatives to prevent illness rather than reacting to illness and treating with prescription drugs, the world would be a healthier place.

The truth is, most people are not aware how good their body is actually designed to feel. This is where enzyme therapy comes into play. For most healthy individuals, our bodies naturally produce an optimal amount of enzymes until we reach our mid- to late-twenties. As we know, some people in their forties may be healthier than someone in their twenties. This can be a result of lifestyle choices, which can effect enzyme production from person to person.

So what are enzymes and why are they vital to your health? Enzymes are biocatalysts or proteins necessary for nearly 3000-4000 of the chemical reactions within our body that are associated with metabolic functions, digestion, detoxification, healthy immune system functioning, growth and natural healing. What does this ultimately mean? It means enzymes help other things work throughout the body. People over the age of 30 have an increased likelihood of enzyme deficiency, which may lead to greater chances of health issues and illnesses.

When people think of enzymes, they most often think digestion. However, there are two different types of enzymes: digestive enzymes and systemic enzymes. Digestive enzymes are taken with a meal and help support overall digestive health by breaking down the food a person eats while also helping to improve nutrient absorption.

Many people are enzyme deficient and do not even know it. According to the National Institute of Health, "60 to 70 million people in America suffer from some type of digestive disorder. People who suffer from poor digestive health are commonly linked to low energy, excessive gas, poor skin health, joint pain, inflammation, weight-gain, weak immune system, heartburn and bloating following meals" {9}. Whether a person is looking to improve their digestive health or may be avoiding certain foods that commonly aggravate the gastrointestinal tract, implementing a well-balanced digestive enzyme complex ensure the body is properly breaking down fats, carbohydrates, proteins into small substrates that can be utilized for energy production throughout the day.

Much different than the role of a digestive enzyme is a systemic enzyme. Systemic enzymes work to support the body as a whole. They are most notably knows for their five main functions: natural anti-inflammatory, anti-fibrin, blood cleansing, immune system modulating and virus fighting. When considering a systemic enzyme supplement, it is important to look at the proprietary blend and delivery system. In order to ensure maximum absorption of activity, an enteric-coated delivery system is ideal which will protect the enzyme activity until the optimal time of release. The enteric-coated delivery system allows it to get past the stomach and into the small intestine without losing enzyme activity, which allows for better absorption.

Proteolytic enzymes or "protein eating enzymes" are the first line of defense against body wide inflammation, which may spread throughout the body to all major organs. Inflammation is a reaction by the immune system to an irritation which often results in pain, swelling or tenderness. Conventional medicine still tends to use pharmaceutical drugs such as ibuprofen and naproxen to reduce inflammation. However, synthetic drugs have many side effects, both minor and severe, that often hinder long-term use in many people. A well-balanced Systemic Enzyme blend will naturally replenish the many enzymes the body uses to fight inflammation and aid in the repair of damaged tissue.

Did you know that nearly all injuries and operations result in inflammatory reactions and build-up of excess scar tissue which causes pain and swelling? It is a natural protective response to injuries and trauma on a cellular level. However, if the inflammation is not resolved ore reduced in the acute stage, it can become a chronic inflammatory problem. When caring for injuries and during recovery following an operation, "it is important to apply medications for reducing the swelling and anti-inflammatory as well as fibrinolytic agents. If possible, such treatment should produce no adverse effects and should further the healing process of the organism". A safe and effective Systemic Enzyme formula, like Innerzyme's Pain & Inflammation Blend, offers a natural solution for post-operative scar tissue, inflammation, and pain following sports injuries and surgery whether recent or fifteen plus years ago.

In addition to it's anti-fibrin properties, systemic enzymes are also known for their ability to cleanse the blood of excess fibrin and exogenous material. Cleaner blood means better nutrient absorption and improved circulation. So how do these toxins and fibrin get into the blood in the first place? The organs and cells in our bodies dispose of these materials in our blood, which can cause clots, poor circulation, blood thickening and other health issues.

How about immune system support and the ability to fight off viruses? Systemic enzymes assist the body to balance the immune system and restore a steady state to the body. A low functioning immune system means the body is more susceptible to disease. However, an extremely high functioning immune system will often create antibodies that attach the tissues within the body such as with autoimmune diseases or arthritis. Supplementation of a well-balanced systemic enzyme may help regulate the immune system and eat away at those antibodies that are attacking the body's tissue creating a disease state within the body.

When it comes to viruses, protein cell walls build up around a virus and then bond together and replicate to cause harm throughout the body. The body knows what the body needs and these harmful protein walls are definitely not needed. The good thing about enzymes is they already know what protein to leave alone and what "foreign" protein to attack and eat away in order to inhibit the replication of the virus.

Oftentimes, you may find yourself with a few extra pounds of weight and feeling sluggish, stressed, and sometimes even depressed. Are you experiencing these post-holiday health blues? Keep reading to find out how to improve your health and reverse the negative effects the holiday season had on you.

Use food as medicine and approach eating in a mindful way. What is mindful eating? Mindful eating is not a diet or meal plan; instead, it's an emerging approach to health that fosters an awareness of what is going on in your body and mind. It encourages you to become aware of your emotional and physiological motivations to eat. By engaging in mindful eating, you are better able to balance what you eat, the way you eat and why you eat.

Here are three steps to get you started on the path to mindful eating:

Tune into physical characteristics of food - Tuning in to the physical characteristics of food involve using three of your senses: smell, taste and sight. With smell, you take in the aroma of the food. Make note of how it smells, is it a pleasant smell? With taste, make note of how it tastes in your mouth and whether it satisfies your taste buds. Notice how it feels in your mouth and whether you enjoy the texture. With sight, how does it look? Is it appealing to you? Use your mind's eye to envision seeing yourself enjoying what you eat.

Tune into repetitive habits and the process of eating - Notice your daily eating patterns. Take note of what times of the day you eat and what activities you are doing that may contribute to mindless eating. These include watching television while you eat, eating at your desk while writing emails, or standing over the sink shoving food into your mouth. Also take notice of whom else is present while eating and what they might be eating; sometimes we like company and eat just because the other person is eating or is present.

Tune into mindless eating triggers - There are certain habits, activities, places, emotions and people that can trigger your eating habits and cause you to eat when you are not even aware of it. You must strive to become aware of what prompts you to eat. Take a deep look at your physical, emotional and environmental triggers. If you know how to recognize your triggers, then you can better anticipate them and catch yourself before you plunge and maybe even begin to change your habits.

Mindful eating is a long-term commitment and takes lots of practice. The main key to this approach is observation. You must first learn to observe your body cues, such as hunger, satiety and energy level. Second, you must observe your psychological state by being aware of your thoughts and emotional triggers. You will get lots of information by observing your mind and your body.

Practice being in the moment; this is easier said than done since most of us run on autopilot much of the time. Sometimes it's easier to fall back on habit or routine rather than being in the moment. Habit and routine take the enjoyment and excitement out of everything and leave you feeling empty and numb. People often eat in an effort to fill the emptiness, however mindless eating only adds to the emptiness. When you are in the moment, you are more apt to notice things as they are happening. Furthermore, you are more aware of how your food tastes, smells, feels in your mouth, and whether it satisfies your hunger or leaves you feeling bloated and sluggish. Practice being in the moment by avoiding eating in front of the television, while driving, or while engaging in other activities and multitasking.

Mind your environment. Create a mindful environment to avoid a toxic environment. Mindful eating environments include those that do not include distractions, are comfortable and promote mindful eating.

Learning and practicing mindful eating will put you on the path to improved health and wellness for the rest of your life. You'll experience increased energy levels, weight loss or maintenance, and an overall sense of peace with food.

CHAPTER 14

YOUR COLON IS VITAL TO YOUR OVERALL HEALTH

Good health depends not only on what goes into your body, but also on what comes out of it. All too often, we underestimate the vital importance of a healthy, properly-functioning colon, and only pay attention if we experience diarrhea or constipation. The reality is that constipation isn't a disease itself, but a symptom of something wrong with the gut. The good news is that, while constipation can be an indication of a more serious problem, it's usually possible to get the colon back on track simply by what you put in your mouth.

The colon is the first four to five feet of the large intestine; it empties into the rectum, which transports stool (feces) to the anus. The colon takes runny, liquefied food from the small intestine, absorbing most of the water and some nutrients, and turns it into solid stool. Water absorption depends on how much time the stool spends in the colon. If it passes through too quickly, it results in watery diarrhea. More commonly, if it stays too long, it becomes dry and hard, and difficult to pass. There can be underlying medical reasons for this, including certain diseases and conditions, advanced age, pregnancy, irritable bowel syndrome, and the effects of prescription or over-the-counter medications, but the primary cause for many Americans is simply poor diet and lack of exercise.

The colon depends on fiber, a substance it cannot digest, to keep everything moving smoothly. Soluble fiber, which dissolves in water, forms a soft gel in the bowel, while non-soluble fiber bulks up the stool and makes it softer and easier to pass. Fiber is found primarily in fruits, vegetables and whole grains, but most Americans eat only a small percentage of the daily recommended amount. Incorporating more fiber-rich foods, and using fiber supplements such as psyllium, will help stools pass easily through the colon.

If the diet has been lacking in fiber for some time, a more intensive plan is often recommended to cleanse the colon and restore it to health. It's not a good idea to use chemical laxatives, especially habitually, as the colon can become dependent on them and become unable to move stools on its own. More natural methods include fiber-intensive diets, a series of dietary supplements, or irrigation with fluid. Once the colon has been cleansed, it should be kept healthy with a fiber-rich diet, enhanced with dietary fiber supplements if necessary, plenty of water, and exercise. Foods and supplements rich in probiotics - the "good bacteria" necessary for nutrient absorption - should also be part of the diet.

The frequency of bowel movements depends on the individual, but the clinical definition of constipation includes fewer than three bowel movements per week, along with hard or lumpy stools, straining to pass stools, or a feeling of still "having to go" after a bowel movement. Hard stools can also cause hemorrhoids or anal fissures. The appearance of the stool is a clue to what's going on inside: it should be medium-brown and almost odorless, and should not be yellow, grey, green, too dark, sticky, or pencil-thin, which can indicate bowel obstruction. The colon is one of the most important organs in your body, and its condition is vital to your overall health.

There are a number of ways to cleanse the colon. Some may seem intrusive while some may be as simple as eating healthy foods and exercising. For those who are considering to jumpstart into healthy living and begin by cleansing the colon, you may consider the following remedies:

Eat a healthy diet. You can start by eating less food that is high in fat, sugar, and processed flour, particularly fast foods. Instead, you should eat large quantities of fruits, steamed vegetables, and foods high in fiber such as cereals and brans.

Also, you may want to consider an enema or colon hydrotherapy. Both procedures involve the introduction of water into the colon through the rectum. However, these procedures are different from each other. An enema only gets to clean the lower part of the colon while a colonic procedure is able to cleanse the entire colon. And contrary to what some might think, a colonic procedure is not at all messy.

But if you are still hesitant to try out colonics, you may try taking herbal cleansing supplements. But these supplements may not be as efficient in cleansing the colon compared to colonic irrigations.

Another oral remedy that is commonly used is laxative. Laxatives may work similarly like herbal cleansing supplements. However, laxatives are known to have a lot of side-effects, mostly due to the fact that people use this remedy inappropriately. Keep in mind that anything that is in done or taken in excess is harmful.

There are also oxygen-based cleansers which are believed to be able to reduce the accumulated toxic wastes into liquid or gas form. This type of cleanser is believed to work not only in the colon but it is believed to work in the entire system.

One of the many benefits of colon cleanse is the prevention of harmful diseases. During the process of cleansing, all the unwanted materials and wastes are eliminated from the body. This results to the treatment of chronic fatigue syndrome and weak immune system. Furthermore, the digestive system is naturally restored, which is important in treating some disorders related to digestion. For instance, the risk of having constipation, diarrhea and stomach upset is reduced.

Colon cleanse also helps you feel more energetic. As toxins and free radicals are accumulated in the body, essential nutrients are not properly absorbed and inappropriate nutrient absorption results to fatigue and lack of energy. With a clean intestinal track, all the essential nutrients are properly used in the body, resulting to more energy and healthier body.

Other benefits of colon cleanse also include keeping the skin glowing and healthy, improving the circulation of blood and enhancing alertness and mental balance. According to research, cleansing also helps in losing weight.

Whichever remedy you may choose, don't ever start without proper diagnosis and advise from a healthcare professional. Moreover, the remedies mentioned above must be used in moderato and upon advice only. Again, anything done or taken in excess is harmful.

CHAPTER 15

LIVING A HEALTHY LIFESTYLE IMPROVES YOUR MIND, BODY AND SPIRIT

Living a healthy life style naturally calls for a healthy body, free from disease and illnesses. It also means that you enjoy a positive outlook about your life, the people in it, and the world.

A healthy lifestyle is one full of energy, without constant stress about aches and pains, and what tomorrow will bring. It's about living in a healthy body, and enjoying the world around you.

What will one get out of healthy living? Just a longer life expectancy, a stronger immunity system, lesser risks to life-threatening diseases-basically a sound mind and body. It is needless to say that choosing this way of life brings about a lot of life-changing benefits.

Living a healthy lifestyle is important and will ultimately prevent acute and chronic diseases. This is quiet easy to achieve as you need not have to take all kinds of supplements or spend hours working out at a gym. All it takes is some independent thinking such as separating the truth from non-truth on current literature and advice.

You cannot change your lifestyle over-night and expect a miracle the following day. This is something you have to do by taking small steps at a time and setting goals for yourself. Once you have achieved one goal, then move onto the next goal and so you go and eventually living a healthy lifestyle will become second nature to you.

A good place to begin and one of the most important factors is eating correctly. Make sure you are following a well-balanced diet that contains loads of fruit and fresh vegetables, whole grains and that you are getting the required amount of vitamins and minerals daily. Avoid gaining weight try and maintain your ideal weight. Don't eat junk food or drink fizzy drinks as these are fat packers. If you are unsure about what foods to eat and how much to eat there are excellent books as well as loads of info on the net.

Another very important way to live a healthy lifestyle is doing daily exercises. This does not mean that you must run out and join a health club, all you have to do is go for long walks, get out and about as physical exercise is not every ones cup of tea. A colon cleanse is also excellent as this type of cleansing eliminates all the toxic waste which makes one feel sluggish.

Everyday modern living suits most people and is also convenient, but detrimental to our health as we eat far too many processed foods and not enough healthy foods. Due to this factor people around the world are fast developing conditions such as diabetes, hypertension, heart disease and various other diseases.

Parents should teach their children from an early age to live a healthy lifestyle and these children will become well balanced healthy kids. Not only will they be healthy in body, but they will also have healthy minds as medical science has proved this time and again. Does it not make 100% sense to rather live a lifestyle of health and happiness as opposed to an unhealthy life and be sickly and miserable?

In order to stay hale and hearty, it is very important to maintain a healthy lifestyle, for all individuals, at all ages. Living such a life means, one has to be deliberately conscious about the fact that whatever foods he eats and the things he performs should not cause any harm to his mind, spirit and body. If one can maintain it, then he will be able to lower the risks of suffering from severe medical conditions, like obesity, high blood pressure and diabetes.

There are several ways, by means of which you can improve your lifestyle. Firstly, to live a healthy lifestyle, you need to change your eating habits. You need to conscious about what type and how much food you are consuming and in what manner the food has been prepared. Cut down the intake of fried and spicy foodstuff and replace it with fresh vegetables, fruits and grains. It is healthier to grill or steam your food, since this will help to preserve the natural minerals and vitamins, which are present in the food.

The second advice that you need to keep in mind, is that to live a healthy lifestyle you need to reduce the consumption of artificial beverages, tea, coffee and soda. It is always better for you, to drink at least 8 glasses of plain water daily, to avoid dehydration as well as to flush out the toxic waste from your body. You can also mix water with electrolytes, especially during hot sultry days.

The third advice is to exercise daily. This will not only help you to live a healthy lifestyle but will also help you to enjoy a happy life. Exercises do not mean that you have to perform strenuous activities. It means you need to keep yourself active and this can be accomplished by simple activities, like swimming, walking and bicycling. You can even join a local gym or can perform free hand exercises or yoga at home. Exercises are good for your body, since they help to increase blood circulations and will keep you fit, strong and healthy.

The fourth important suggestion is to free oneself from addictive behaviors, which are harmful to your mind, spirit and body, like alcohol consumption and smoking. This will not only enhance your health conditions, but also help you to live a healthy lifestyle.

The fifth advice is that you should always try to maintain a happy and positive viewpoint. You can join clubs, meditation or yoga centers or participate in various activities, as these things will not only improve your life but will also keep your spirit and mind in high spirits, away from stress and tension.

Develop These Simple Habits and Start Living a Healthy Lifestyle

Choosing to live a healthy lifestyle doesn't always mean submitting yourself to fancy exercises and depriving yourself of foods. There are simple habits that you can start to develop to improve the quality of your health. These are inexpensive and easy to do.

You can start by regularly drinking at least 8 glasses of water a day. Depending on your level of activity each day and the climate where you live, you may be required to drink more. But eight glasses are the minimum and following this simple requirement helps a lot in flushing out unwanted elements from your body. If you can't live without soda, limit your intake to one can per week. There's little nutrition you can get from this beverage and they're full of sugar and calories which can only worsen any existing illnesses you have.

More and more people are diagnosed with diabetes each day. This is because of the proliferation of unhealthy sweet foods in the market today. If you have a sweet tooth, try to limit your sugar intake to a reasonable amount to avoid developing diabetes and adding unwanted pounds to your weight. If your resolve to maintain a healthy lifestyle is strong enough, you should be able to cut it off completely. You can add more antioxidants in your diet by eating plenty of fruits and vegetables. As you know, antioxidants play an important role in keeping the cells in your body healthy. They're proven to prevent development of certain kinds of cancer and heart diseases. So, snack on organic produce instead of getting your hands on a cookie jar every time you feel hungry in between meals.

Stressing yourself over some things can wear your mind and body out. It is important that you know how to give it a rest so you can recharge and invigorate your sense once more. Being stressed can give out a negative vibe and this can harm your goal towards healthy living. Doing physical exercises is a good way of refreshing your mind and body. This also gives you a chance to take your mind off other things and focus only in keeping your mind and body fit. If you can't find time to go to a gym, a 30-minute walk each day will do the trick. If your office and grocery is only a walking distance, leave your car in the garage and work up a sweat by walking to work. Not only are you slowly improving your health but you are also saving up on gas money and helping the environment free from pollutants.

You have heard your mom say this to you and you will hear it again. Make the habit of brushing and flossing at least two times a day. You may have overlooked its importance but your teeth are a big part of your health. Through a person's teeth, one can tell what kind of lifestyle he is keeping. The bacteria that are left in your mouth can give you all kind of diseases. It doesn't take much to brush and floss every time you wake up and before you hit the bed every night.

CHAPTER 16

SEVEN HABITS TO LIVE HEALTHY

There are many ways to keep resolutions for a healthy lifestyle; putting a price tag on your failure (make a bet with someone and be ready to pay if you don't stick to a plan), making small goals instead of focusing solely on the end results, and finding yourself an accountability partner who can help challenge you on the days you lose your motivation.

There are 7 habits that people who live healthy lifestyles all have in common. These habits involve self-mastery as well as mastery over our interactions with others and our perception of the world.

Pick your battles: We are all inundated with potentially stressful situations every day however there is a brief moment where we have the unique human ability to choose our response. Unfortunately, we have all been conditioned throughout our lives to react in certain ways to certain circumstances, and by reacting with conditioned responses, we give up our precious ability to choose the outcome.

For example, if someone is rude or inflammatory to us, our conditioned response would generally be to respond back, at the very least, with annoyance and sometimes even anger. Instead of giving in to this conditioned reaction, we can choose to not let it bother us, or even better, we can choose to understand and forgo the tension. If we can choose positive, or at the very least, neutral responses it has the power to bring us closer to our goals and increase the boundaries of what we can control. On the other hand, poorly chosen responses, or conditioned responses that are merely thoughtless reactions, will likely bring about negative consequences and shrink our scope of influence. This generally leads to feeling more out of control over your lot in life when, in reality, our responses often shape our perceptions and, indeed, even determine success or failure.

Take responsibility for your health: Poor health and disease are at an all-time high and many of us assume this as a normal part of aging. Many people accept the burden of their poor health and the compromised quality of life that comes along with it as something that just "is" instead of something that can be controlled. They put themselves into the hands of doctors and pharmaceutical companies instead of taking an active role in their own self-care. This is a prime, but unfortunate example of a conditioned reaction.

Instead of accepting poor health or chronic disease as your fate, be proactive by challenging the notion that you are a helpless victim and take responsibility for your health by carving out and living a healthier lifestyle.

Create and visualize your "end game".: Get clear on what it is you really want. Take time to visualize what it is you really want to achieve whether it is balanced health, more money, to be more organized, or creating an entirely new life, allowing yourself to really be clear about exactly what you want in your life will help you create a plan to get there. Writing this end game down or creating a board in which you have cut out pictures of your ideal life will allow you to keep it fresh and clear in your mind.

Once you have your end game expressed you will be able to make smaller goals that ultimately will help you reach your desired result. Taking stock of your smaller achievements will show you how much further you have to go in making your goal. Also, having a clear understanding of your goals allows you to make smarter decisions that are more supportive of achieving them.

Begin with Your Health in Mind: The health you have as you grow older will be exactly the culmination of all of your health choices up to that point. If you wish to be physically active, mentally sharp and full of energy in your old age, the decisions you make today and every day after should be heavily influenced by this desired result.

Poor health and disease did not happen overnight. While you may not feel as if your health is compromised, your daily habits may still be promoting disease through chronic inflammation and acid forming diet, and if they are, they will eventually catch up with you. It can be extremely difficult but luckily never impossible to reverse the damage caused by unhealthy habits which is why the lifestyle you choose today should be lived with the best possible health choices to positively affect your health in your golden years.

Get your priorities straight

There are only 24 hours in a single day and if you don't manage your time wisely, many of the things you hope to accomplish will never get done. Mastering the first two habits will teach you to commit yourself to action and getting clear on your desired end result but you must then have a clear understanding and the discipline to match in order to prioritize the actions that will help you achieve your goals. Without this, you'll end up wasting time on frivolous activities and your goals will become much harder to achieve. Luckily, by taking small steps to increase your productivity (setting timers for tasks, uninstalling "Angry Birds", and creating a definitive schedule for Facebook, Twitter and other social networks), you will find it gets easier to stick with priorities that really matter.

Make your health your number one priority: Certain aspects of living a healthy lifestyle are often thought of as restrictive, time consuming, or just plain difficult. If you attempt to follow a lifestyle that is too restrictive and complicated, you will certainly become burned out and frustrated, and will more than likely return to your old unhealthy habits sooner than later. This is not inevitable, however and full preventable if you invest your time and effort wisely by focusing on adding in healthier activities and nutrition instead of on taking away the negative aspects of your routines. Slowly, the good will crowd out the bad.

For example, let's say you hate the gym. You decide to embark on a healthy lifestyle so you sign up for a gym membership. You go and buy trainers, clothing, all the bells and whistles of what going to the gym entails. You even go for a week, two, maybe even a few months. Slowly you remember that you do not like running on a treadmill, can't stand waiting in line for the weight machines or jockeying for a position You cut back your time at the gym, at first by 10 minutes then by a day until one day you realize you have stopped going. What you really do like is to be outside. Instead of going to the gym, make time to take a 20-minute walk outside after or during lunch or after dinner and pick a place to walk that you love. If you like shopping, going window shopping is a great way to get your exercise and figure out what you'll buy when you lose those 5 pounds. You work at a desk all day so why not create a standing work station or bring a pedal bike for under your desk. Building in 5 minute stretch breaks for every 20 minutes of work, reaching down and touching your toes while picking up the kids clothes off the floor, parking your car further away from the entrance from the mall or taking the stairs those three flights up to your apartment instead of the lift are fantastic ways to build in exercise and not have to step foot in a gym.

With food, instead of going cold turkey on all your favorite foods, perhaps you choose to add in a green smoothie or juice, use spinach instead of romaine lettuce in your wraps. You try one new vegetable or fruit a week. You commit to one meatless meal in a week. Then, you start to notice that you are getting more satisfied including foods that you don't have as much room as you normally would for junk food. There are many ways to make eating healthy delicious so you never feel deprived. Being healthy does not have to be painful.

Cultivate a win/win scenario: We all naturally use

personal gain as a strong motivation in life. Because of this fact most problems or challenges that affects others is best resolved through a solution that benefits everyone involved.

Many people only care about "what's in it for them" and pay little attention to the effects that their decisions have on others. These people are limiting themselves, often without realizing, because it is far more difficult to achieve goals without the help and support of others. In some cases, even impossible. Eventually, in time, even these people realize they need help from those around them, but because they have a tendency to be self-centered and imposing, they are unlikely to get it.

Look for a win/win with your health: With the many distracting and negative influences of our society, it often requires a lot of discipline and motivation to achieve and maintain good health. Having the support of the people around you make it significantly easier. In the same regard, if you allow your healthy lifestyle to impose on the lives of others, you might find they resist your healthy lifestyle changes or risk alienating them which makes your pursuit of a healthy lifestyle more difficult.

Your family members tend to be your most important relationships and have the most significant potential for providing support and it is important to have them on your side. Better health is an obvious win for yourself, but your effort to achieve it may be a source of contention among your family members. However, if you handle the situation intelligently, your ambition for better health has the potential to be a big win for your family as well.

Understand to be understood: Stubbornness and an unwillingness to at least acknowledge another person's viewpoint is the number one reason many relationships erode.

When someone opposes an opinion that you hold strongly, it's often a natural reaction to push your opinion harder. This is often met with further opposition and can cause a downward spiral that leads to an ugly argument or even a damaged relationship. The only way to avoid this situation and turn it into a productive conversation is to make an emphatic effort to understand the opposing point of view before arguing against it. In many cases, you'll either find that the opposition was based on a misunderstanding, or you'll learn something new.

Seeking First to Understand Better Health

In pursuit of better health, it is a virtual certainty you will come across many varied differing viewpoints and suggestions, even from doctors and health care professionals. Many opinions will be diametrically opposed to each other. The profit based motivations of big business tend to make these different viewpoints even worse, often fostering more confusion with every new diet book published. Health related opinions tend to be debated with great passion, and as such, it greatly increases the need for effective and considerate communication.

Harmonize to synergize: Synergy is often a result of the previous two habits. When all parties are focused on finding a solution that will benefit everyone, and when each varied opinion is taken into account, the result is usually a series of creative possibilities and opportunities that would have never been conceived independently.

Creating synergy in your health: The human body is a complex organism and there are still many questions still unanswered by modern medicine. Many health conditions, as a result, may seem impossible to resolve. A one sided approach to resolving any health condition is never as effective as the treating the condition with a synergistic approach. By listening to all the angles given by the varied opinions of health care professionals, doctors, even family and friends we often open the door to new ideas and opportunities for improving or, indeed, even renewing our well-being.

Stay sharp, focused, and maintain balance: Being

effective is being able to make intentional progress towards an established objective. The previous six habits provide the tools you need to promote balance and development within the physical, spiritual, mental and social aspects of your life, and in turn, become a more complete and effective person. Staying sharp and focused is about continuing your growth by maintaining this balance.

Keeping our bodies healthy is key in our ability to enjoy life to the fullest. Being spiritually at ease by having a firm grasp on our values and inspirations allows us to guide our lives in the direction of what we wish to experience. Staying mentally sharp and expanding our knowledge increases our ability to understand and recognize our spirituality and to keep our lives on track with the direction it provides. Finally, social interaction is one of the most satisfying aspects of life and gives us a feeling of belonging, provides fulfillment, and in turn, promotes better health.

CONCLUSION

There are no concrete answers on how to live longer, healthier, or even safer. The only way is to practice living a healthy lifestyle. The goals that we set, need to start somewhere. You have to start by changing routines that may damper or set back your goals. Your body's organs need to me exercised or used the correct way so they are able to grow the correct way.

Having an unhealthy lifestyle can cause many unwanted physical and mental problems. Most people don't realize how much strain is on your mind and body when you don't have the right level of hormones and vitamins in your body, which accompany a healthy lifestyle.

Many people think these diseases and sicknesses are inherited and that there is nothing they can do to prevent or heal them. This is not true in most cases! Watching what you eat and getting the right amount of exercise will make you feel much better than taking some kind of pill for your problem. For example someone with high blood-pressure or high sugar can take medications that can help them to control their disease but what many of them don't know is that if they did regular cardiovascular exercise and ate healthier foods they probably wouldn't even have to take the medications and would also feel great!

Most people want to live a healthy lifestyle but they don't have the right tools to get started. They also don't maintain the self-motivation it takes to be persistent enough to stick to a healthy living pattern. The first thing to do is to decide what your goals are. Once you have come up with your goals then you have accomplished the first step to your healthy lifestyle!

The main point to remember is that the only way to get your healthy lifestyle is to keep on trying every day. Eventually your lifestyle changes become second nature. In other words, after you become accustomed to your lifestyle changes they will become a way of life instead of something you are making yourself do to feel good.

There are many diet and exercise plans out there. You must keep in mind that many of these are based on people who want to make money and they are not good for you! You must find the plans that are best for you. Fad diets and exercise plans that wear you out are most likely not the right choices.

One of the best tips for maintaining your healthy

lifestyle is to not let anything you do set you back. Give yourself breaks and when you eat something that is not on your diet plan or you skip a day exercising. Also, with every accomplishment you make give yourself credit. Everyone is human. Once you achieve your new healthy lifestyle you will be sorry you didn't do it a long time ago. You will feel like a new person.

Living a healthier lifestyle takes dedication. A lot of enjoyments in life are hazardous to your healthy lifestyle. Smoking, drinking, drugs, the night life, foods, or even your job duties. It comes down to every action during your day. From what we put in to what we produce. Not only may we consume fatty or unhealthy foods, but the mind takes in everything as well. You brain is a powerful organ that needs to be taken care of. We need to fill our lifestyle with healthier images. Starting from a child, we notice everything. A son follows his father, watches, then mimics his actions. We need to produce healthier results for other to notice. A healthy lifestyle needs to be a daily activity. Everyone has a different idea of how to live a healthier lifestyle. Everyone has different beliefs.

You probably have heard of anti-inflammatory medications. But did you know that there is a relationship that exists between inflammation and diet? Indeed, there is such a thing as an anti-inflammatory diet which consists of foods that prevent onset of inflammations.

The food we eat can affect inflammation in an unpredictably complex manner. The best advice to follow is to avoid "pro-inflammatory foods" or foods that increase inflammation, and take in more of anti-inflammatory food sources. This means taking less of saturated fats found in meats, eggs, and dairy products which are rich in inflammation-promoting arachidonic acid, while taking more or low fat milk, lean meat, fish and vegetables. It is also important to avoid taking in too much sugar as it is not only related to inflammation but to obesity and many other chronic diseases as well.

The benefits of maintaining a healthy diet free of pro-inflammatory compounds do not only free you from the risk of developing inflammation and conditions that go with it, but it also provides long term benefits. You will eventually realize how a good anti-inflammatory diet can make your skin look younger, remove the allergy symptoms, make your joints feel better, and give you an overall healthy feeling.

Omega-3 fatty acids in fish oil are one of the most important aspects in a healthy, anti-inflammatory diet. These essential fatty acids are very potent anti-inflammatory agents that can protect and relieve you from all forms of inflammation. You can get your daily dose of omega 3 fish oils through intake of adequate amounts of fish and seafood, or take a regular dose of fish oil supplements. Make sure to consult with your nutritionist or doctor regarding appropriate dosage.

Aside from the strong relationship between inflammation and diet, research studies also suggest the importance of leading healthy lifestyle habits such as exercising regularly, maintaining an ideal weight, minimizing stress, and avoidance of smoking and alcohol.

The foods that we eat help maintain that healthy body. Your lifestyle starts with the amount of sleep we get each night to the exercise your body needs. The types of body everyone has needs different amounts. Everyone is created different. Food is the source of your energy. What you consume is what you produce. Vitamins are an excellent source of nutrition to replenish what your body lacks to absorb. Do you consider yourself healthy? Are there areas in your lifestyle that need to be removed or altered to reach your goals?

Good health does not only involve being free of disease. A healthy person keeps their mind and body in great shape, both of which can contribute to a better lifestyle. There are many ways of improving and maintaining your health

Living in a clean environment also helps improve

your health. It is a proven fact that germs that cause illness thrive best in unhygienic surroundings. Clear your home, school or office desk from dust, dampness and congestion, and keep doing this to make it a good habit. Do your best to live in areas that have fresh air circulating, clean dry storage spaces for perishable foodstuff and always clean your environment regularly. Also remember to exercise personal hygiene so your body will be unsuitable to host disease-causing germs.

In short, optimum nutrition is about providing the body cells and tissues with the vitamins and minerals they require to function to their best ability. If this lifestyle of optimum nutrition is applied from an early age, it is likely to be your best guarantee for a long and healthy life.

You should, of course, consult with your health care professional before starting any diet, exercise, or supplementation program. The information provided in this article is for informational purposes only and is not intended as a substitute for advice from your health care provider. Just make sure that you do your own health research as well...it will be a learning experience for which your body will thank you with improved health if you diligently fuel it with optimum nutrition on a daily basis.

Improved immunity and resistance to disease,

prevention of conditions such as heart disease and diabetes, a longer life-expectancy, and a higher quality of life are just a few of the many benefits of living a healthy lifestyle. As technology has made our lives easier, it has also made us lazier and more sedentary than our ancestors. For this reason, it is more important to develop and maintain a healthy lifestyle. So what can you do to be healthier?

Contrary to popular belief, living healthy does not have to be an exceptional challenge. If you are interested in developing a healthier balance with respect to your physical and mental condition, you only need to make a few minor changes over time. Eventually, you will be in a position where you are eating healthy, exercising regularly, and maintaining an ideal work-life balance.

Ultimately, just a few small changes to your routine can help you achieve a healthier and happier lifestyle. And remember, you don't need to make all these changes at once. Instead, you should try to make a long term plan and introduce gradual changes over time so that you don't feel like you're completely revamping your life.

DISCLAIMER

The information contained within this eBook is strictly for educational purposes. If you wish to apply ideas contained in this eBook, you are taking full responsibility for your actions.

The author has made every effort to ensure the accuracy of the information within this book was correct at time of publication. The author does not assume and hereby disclaims any liability to any party for any loss, damage, or disruption caused by errors or omissions, whether such errors or omissions result from accident, negligence, or any other cause. (DIET, Intermittent fasting)

DO NOT GO YET;
ONE LAST THING TO DO

If you enjoyed this book or found it useful, I'd be very grateful if you'd post a short review on it. Your support really does make a difference and I read all the reviews personally so I can get your feedback and make this book even better.

Thanks again for your support!